Copyright © 2o20 by Cameron Bartley -All rights reserved.

No part of this publication may be reproduced, distributed, or transmitted in any form or by any means, including photocopying, recording, or other electronic or mechanical methods, without the prior written permission of the publisher, except in the case of brief quotations embodied in reviews and certain other non-commercial uses permitted by copyright law.

This Book is provided with the sole purpose of providing relevant information on a specific topic for which every reasonable effort has been made to ensure that it is both accurate and reasonable. Nevertheless, by purchasing this Book you consent to the fact that the author, as well as the publisher, are in no way experts on the topics contained herein, regardless of any claims as such that may be made within. It is recommended that you always consult a professional prior to undertaking any of the advice or techniques discussed within.This is a legally binding declaration that is considered both valid and fair by both the Committee of Publishers Association and the American Bar Association and should be considered as legally binding within the United States.

CONTENTS

INTRODUCTION 6
APPETIZERS AND SIDE DISHES 8
1. Bacon Wrapped Asparagus 8
2. Air Fried Green Tomatoes(1) 8
3. Garlic & Parmesan Bread Bites 8
4. Coriander Artichokes(1) 8
5. Shrimp With Spices 8
6. Goat Cheese & Pancetta Bombs 9
7. Kale And Walnuts(1) 9
8. Beef Enchilada Dip 9
9. Jicama Fries(3) 9
10. Parsley Mushroom Pilaf 10
11. Bok Choy And Butter Sauce(2) 10
12. Cherry Farro 10
13. Baked Artichoke Hearts 10
14. Homemade Chicken Thighs 11
15. Polenta Sticks 11
16. Healthy Asparagus Potatoes 11
17. Party Macaroni Quiche With Greek Yogurt 11
18. Baked Sweet Potatoes 12
19. Homemade Cod Fingers 12
20. Potato Chips With Creamy Lemon Dip 12
21. Mashed Squash 12
22. Roasted Radishes With Brown Butter, Lemon, And Radish Tops 13
23. Spinach And Artichokes Sauté 13
24. Sesame Garlic Chicken Wings 13
25. Winter Vegetables With Herbs 13
26. Chili Lime Sweet Potatoes 14
27. Crispy Zucchini Sticks 14
28. Sweet Carrot Puree 14
29. Cheddar & Prosciutto Strips 15
30. Parmesan Cauliflower 15
31. Kale And Walnuts(2) 15
32. Cheesy Garlic Biscuits 15
33. Homemade Prosciutto Wrapped Cheese Sticks ... 16
34. Rosemary Chickpeas 16
35. Bacon & Potato Salad With Mayonnaise 16
36. Tasty Hassel Back Potatoes 16
37. Baked Broccoli 16
38. Crispy Cauliflower Poppers 17
39. Glazed Carrots 17
BREAKFAST RECIPES 18
40. Prosciutto & Mozzarella Crostini 18
41. Egg Florentine With Spinach 18
42. Eggplant Hoagies 18
43. Ham And Cheese Toast 18
44. Stuffed Poblanos 19
45. Healthy Baked Oatmeal 19
46. Savory Cheddar & Cauliflower Tater Tots 20
47. Raspberries Maple Pancakes 20
48. Mozzarella Endives And Tomato Salad 20
49. Quick Mac & Cheese 20
50. Healthy Tofu Omelet 21
51. Chicken & Zucchini Omelet 21
52. Easy Cheesy Breakfast Casserole 21
53. Crustless Broccoli Quiche 21
54. Whole Wheat Carrot Bread 22
55. Parmesan Asparagus 22
56. Pumpkin And Yogurt Bread 22
57. Delicious Baked Omelet 23
58. Banana & Peanut Butter Cake 23
59. Spinach Zucchini Egg Muffins 23
60. Asparagus And Cheese Strata 24
61. Sweet Breakfast Casserole 24
62. Banana Oat Muffins 25
63. Bacon Bread Egg Casserole 25
64. Vanilla Granola 25
65. Chicken Breakfast Sausages 25
66. Baked Peanut Butter Oatmeal 26
67. Potato Egg Casserole 26
68. Smoked Sausage Breakfast Mix 26
69. Spinach & Kale Balsamic Chicken 27
70. Beans And Pork Mix 27
71. Oats, Chocolate Chip, Pecan Cookies 27
72. Egg And Avocado Burrito 28
73. Avocado Oil Gluten Free Banana Bread Recipe 28
74. Smart Oven Baked Oatmeal Recipe 29
75. Chives Salmon And Shrimp Bowls 29
76. Simply Bacon 29
77. Herby Mushrooms With Vermouth 29
78. Crispy Tilapia Tacos 29
LUNCH RECIPES 31
79. Zucchini Stew 31
80. Beef Steaks With Beans 31
81. Easy Italian Meatballs 31
82. Perfect Size French Fries 31
83. Sweet Potato And Parsnip Spiralized Latkes 32
84. Crispy Breaded Pork Chop 32
85. Pumpkin Pancakes 32
86. Lobster Tails 33
87. Roasted Mini Peppers 33
88. Air Fried Steak Sandwich 33
89. Skinny Black Bean Flautas 34

90. Turkey And Mushroom Stew 34
91. Moroccan Pork Kebabs 34
92. Spicy Avocado Cauliflower Toast 35
93. Spanish Chicken Bake 35
94. Barbecue Air Fried Chicken 36
95. Bok Choy And Butter Sauce(1) 36
96. Mushroom Meatloaf 36
97. Eggplant And Leeks Stew 37
98. Garlic Chicken Potatoes 37
99. Turkey-stuffed Peppers 37
100. Fried Whole Chicken 38
101. Seven-layer Tostadas 38
102. Parmesan Chicken Meatballs 38
103. Sweet & Sour Pork 39
104. Pork Stew 39
105. Turkey Meatballs With Manchego Cheese 39
106. Okra Casserole 40
107. Persimmon Toast With Sour Cream & Cinnamon 40
108. Okra And Green Beans Stew 40
109. Air Fried Sausages 40
110. Vegetarian Philly Sandwich 41
111. Coconut Shrimp With Dip 41
112. Kale And Pine Nuts 41
113. Chicken With Veggies And Rice 42
114. Rolled Salmon Sandwich 42
115. Turkey Meatloaf 42
116. Spicy Green Crusted Chicken 42
117. Lamb Gyro 43

DINNER RECIPES **44**
118. Herbed Eggplant 44
119. Lemon Duck Legs 44
120. Shrimp Kebabs 44
121. Delicious Beef Roast With Red Potatoes 45
122. Air Fryer Veggie Quesdillas 45
123. Coconut Crusted Shrimp 45
124. Miso-glazed Salmon 46
125. Couscous Stuffed Tomatoes 46
126. Shrimps, Zucchini, And Tomatoes On The Grill 46
127. Spicy Cauliflower Rice 46
128. Rigatoni With Roasted Broccoli And Chick Peas 47
129. Chargrilled Halibut Niçoise With Vegetables .. 47
130. Marinated Cajun Beef 47
131. Coconut-crusted Haddock With Curried Pumpkin Seeds 48
132. Easy Air Fryed Roasted Asparagus 48
133. Creamy Breaded Shrimp 48
134. Chinese-style Spicy And Herby Beef 49

135. Lemongrass Pork Chops 49
136. Broccoli With Olives 49
137. Artichoke Spinach Casserole 50
138. Beef, Mushrooms And Noodles Dish 50
139. Rice And Tuna Puff 50
140. Creole Beef Meatloaf 51
141. Tex-mex Chicken Quesadillas 51
142. Broccoli Stuffed Peppers 51
143. Indian Meatballs With Lamb 52
144. Pesto & White Wine Salmon 52
145. Air Fryer Buffalo Mushroom Poppers 52
146. Roasted Garlic Zucchini Rolls 53
147. Creamy Tuna Cakes 53
148. Traditional English Fish And Chips 54
149. Pork Chops With Chicory Treviso 54
150. Grilled Tasty Scallops 54
151. Cheesy Shrimp 54
152. Morning Ham And Cheese Sandwich 55
153. Coco Mug Cake 55
154. Cinnamon Pork Rinds 55
155. Smoked Ham With Pears 55
156. Vegetable Cane 56

MEAT RECIPES **57**
157. Cracker Apple Chicken 57
158. Beef Rolls With Pesto & Spinach 57
159. Teriyaki Chicken Thighs With Lemony Snow Peas 57
160. Lemon Mustard Chicken 58
161. Air Fried London Broil 58
162. Citrus Carnitas 58
163. Chicken & Cheese Enchilada 59
164. Spice-coated Steaks With Cucumber And Snap Pea Salad 59
165. Tuscan Air Fried Veal Loin 60
166. Honey Bbq Lamb Chops 60
167. Rosemary Turkey Scotch Eggs 60
168. Parmesan Cajun Pork Chops 61
169. Chicken Thighs With Radish Slaw 61
170. Barbecue Chicken And Coleslaw Tostadas 61
171. Cheesy Pepperoni And Chicken Pizza 62
172. Juicy Spicy Lemon Kebab 62
173. Beef Steak Oregano Fingers 62
174. Beef French Toast 63
175. Cayenne Chicken Drumsticks 63
176. Calf's Liver Golden Strips 63
177. Crispy Cracker Crusted Pork Chops 64
178. Rustic Pork Ribs 64
179. Mom's Meatballs 64

180. Ranch Pork Chops 64
181. Crispy Crusted Chicken 65
182. Flavorful Sirloin Steak 65
183. Meatballs(14) 65
184. Greek Chicken Breast 66
185. Chicken Madeira 66
186. Air Fry Chicken Drumsticks 66
187. Lime-chili Chicken Wings 67
188. Ham Flat Cakes 67
189. Corn Flour Lamb Fries With Red Chili 67
190. Smoky Paprika Pork And Vegetable Kabobs... 67
191. Turkey Grandma's Easy To Cook Wontons 68
192. Grandma's Ground Beef Balls 68
193. Caraway Crusted Beef Steaks 68
194. Chicken Skewers With Corn Salad 69
195. Parmesan Chicken Cutlets 69

FISH & SEAFOOD RECIPES 70
196. Breaded Fish Fillets 70
197. Tomato Garlic Shrimp 70
198. Tuna Sandwich 70
199. Old Bay Crab Cakes 71
200. Rosemary Buttered Prawns 71
201. Crispy Paprika Fish Fillets(1) 71
202. Prawn French Cuisine Galette 71
203. Crispy Salmon With Lemon-butter Sauce 72
204. Basil White Fish 72
205. Baked Tilapia With Garlic Aioli 72
206. Fish Club Classic Sandwich 73
207. Lemon Butter Shrimp 73
208. Cheese Carp Fries 73
209. Basil Salmon With Tomatoes 74
210. Tuna Lettuce Wraps 74
211. Baked Pesto Salmon 74
212. Tasty Parmesan Shrimp 75
213. Crispy Paprika Fish Fillets(2) 75
214. Fish Spicy Lemon Kebab 75
215. Shrimp And Cherry Tomato Kebabs 75
216. Easy Scallops 76
217. Herb Baked Catfish Fillets 76
218. Cajun Catfish Cakes With Cheese 77
219. Spinach & Tuna Balls With Ricotta 77
220. Panko Crab Sticks With Mayo Sauce 77
221. Garlic Butter Shrimp Scampi 78
222. Tasty Tuna Loaf 78
223. Golden Beer-battered Cod 78
224. Parmesan Fish With Pine Nuts 79
225. Citrus Cilantro Catfish 79
226. Salmon Beans & Mushrooms 79
227. Roasted Nicoise Salad 79
228. Baked Scallops 80
229. Buttery Crab Legs 80
230. Cheesy Tilapia Fillets 80
231. Cajun Salmon With Lemon 80
232. Sesame Seeds Coated Fish 81
233. Spicy Halibut 81
234. Simple Lemon Salmon 81

MEATLESS RECIPES 82
235. Mushroom Club Sandwich 82
236. Tofu, Carrot And Cauliflower Rice 82
237. Green Chili Taquitos 82
238. Vegetable And Cheese Stuffed Tomatoes 83
239. Cilantro Roasted Carrots With Cumin Seeds... 83
240. Cheddar & Bean Burritos 83
241. Fried Root Vegetable Medley With Thyme 83
242. Honey-glazed Roasted Veggies 84
243. Cheese With Spinach Enchiladas 84
244. Rosemary Butternut Squash Roast 85
245. Potato Flat Cakes 85
246. Cottage Cheese Fried Baked Pastry 85
247. Roasted Butternut Squash With Maple Syrup 86
248. Teriyaki Tofu 86
249. Crispy Tofu Sticks 86
250. Korean Tempeh Steak With Broccoli 86
251. Cauliflower Rice With Tofu & Peas 87
252. Spicy Thai-style Vegetables 87
253. Spicy Kung Pao Tofu 87
254. Chili Veggie Skewers 88
255. Cottage Cheese And Mushroom Mexican Burritos 88
256. Veg Momo's Recipe 89
257. Gourd French Cuisine Galette 89
258. Paprika Cauliflower 89
259. Russian-style Eggplant Caviar 90
260. Lemony Brussels Sprouts And Tomatoes 90
261. Parmesan Breaded Zucchini Chips 90
262. Okra Flat Cakes 91
263. Potato Fried Baked Pastry 91
264. Zucchini Crisps 91
265. Honey-glazed Baby Carrots 92
266. Grandma´s Ratatouille 92
267. Cabbage Flat Cakes 92
268. Mint French Cuisine Galette 92
269. Banana Best Homemade Croquette 93
270. Onion Rings 93
271. Chili Sweet Potato Fries 93
272. Cheesy Spinach Toasties 93

273. Parmesan Cabbage With Blue Cheese Sauce... 94
SNACKS AND DESSERTS RECIPES 95
274. Vanilla Peanut Butter Cake.. 95
275. Almond Cranberry Muffins....................................... 95
276. Cinnamon Apple Crisp... 95
277. Pita Bread Cheese Pizza.. 96
278. Seafood Turnovers... 96
279. Margherita Pizza.. 96
280. Tasty Jalapeno Poppers 97
281. Deep-dish Giant Double Chocolate Chip Cookie97
282. Cappuccino Blondies... 97
283. Tasty Potato Wedges... 97
284. Italian Rice Balls.. 98
285. Flavorful Coconut Cake 98
286. Strawberries Stew.. 99
287. Coffee Flavored Doughnuts..................................... 99
288. Nutella Banana Pastries... 99
289. Simple Lemon Pie.. 99
290. Buffalo Style Cauliflower 100
291. Spicy Snack Mix... 100
292. Easy Lemon Cheesecake 100
293. Baked Yoghurt 101
294. Easy Blueberry Muffins.. 101
295. Easy Bacon Jalapeno Poppers............................... 101
296. Tasty Broccoli Fritters.. 101
297. Cheesy Baked Potatoes 102
298. Tasty Gingersnap Cookies..................................... 102
299. Almond Flour Blackberry Muffins 103
300. Cheesy Zucchini Tots.. 103

INTRODUCTION

Preparing better food is an energy for everyone most definitely. This has to do with the devices utilized for cooking. Some Utensil causes cooking simpler and quicker while some to don't. Everybody chooses Utensil that prepares food quicker and flavorful. So, it bodes well that Air fryer broiler is one of the kitchen utensils that prepares food quicker and scrumptious. It has picked up prominence throughout the years.

Kalorik Maxx Air fryer stove is in this manner a kitchen apparatus that utilizes convection to course hot air everywhere throughout the prepared nourishment for a decent, more advantageous and flavorful conveyance. Some of the time oil can be utilized however negligible and not obligatory.

The Kalorik Maxx Air fryer stove was likewise modified to utilize a teaspoon of oil to sear nourishments. Nourishments singed with the Air fryer broiler gives comparative taste contrasted with the ones cooked with other weight cookers or burner.

More or less, Kalorik Maxx Air fryer broiler is a little kitchen unit that works like a convection stove. It utilizes air to broil food. Their costs extend in sizes. To warm the air, they utilize electrical components. At the point when the air is hot, it circles this hot air around the food.

Advantages Of Cooking With An Air Fryer Stove

Nourishments cooked with the Kalorik Maxx Air fryer broiler gives comparative taste and are more advantageous contrasted with the ones cooked with other weight cookers or burner. They resemble a little convection broiler. As expressed before, they utilize electrical components to warm the air.

At the point when the air is hot, it courses this hot air around the food. This hot air prepares the food and makes it fresh.

There are numerous advantages gotten from cooking with the Kalorik Maxx Air fryer stove. They are counted beneath.

The Unit Is Anything But Easy To Work With:

Kalorik Maxx Air fryer stove was modified in a unique manner with the end goal that its activity isn't so troublesome. You simply need to set Cooking Time, temperature, put the food and shake the cooking bin few moments while cooking. In the event that you shake the container, it will assist your food with being cooked appropriately.

It Prepares Food Quicker:

The unit prepares food quicker with ideal outcome. The arrangement of coursing the air around with fans, makes it cook nourishments quicker in light of the fact that Air fryer broiler takes few moments to preheat while other cooking units may take as long as 30 minutes to come to pressure.

Cleaning The Air Fryer Stove Isn't Repetitive:

A few people feel disheartened with regards to cleaning their cooking unit. The Kalorik Maxx Air fryer stove makes it not repetitive in light of the fact that you just need to clean the cooking container and dish. With nonstick cooking shower, food isn't typically adhered to the container but instead slides directly off onto your plate. It doesn't require some investment to wash the unit after use.

It Gives Healthier Cooking:

Everybody needs to eat well food to support their prosperity. This utensil can assist you with cooking any fries like solidified fries, chicken wings, onion rings and numerous others. This can be cooked without the utilization of oil. These nourishments are more beneficial because of its low fat and oil content. Like the customary broiler, fries from the Air fryer stove are crispier and more beneficial.

Without futher ado, let's start trying our recipes made for you for your pleaseure in easy cooking!

APPETIZERS AND SIDE DISHES

1. Bacon Wrapped Asparagus

Servings: 4
Cooking Time: 4
Ingredients:
- 20 spears asparagus
- 4 bacon slices
- 1 tbsp olive oil
- 1 tbsp sesame oil
- 1 tbsp brown sugar
- 1 garlic clove, crushed

Directions:
1. Preheat Kalorik Maxx on Air Fry function to 380 F. In a bowl, mix the oils, sugar, and crushed garlic. Separate the asparagus into 4 bunches (5 spears in 1 bunch) and wrap each bunch with a bacon slice. Coat the bunches with the oil mixture. Place them in your Air Fryer basket and fit in the baking tray. Cook for 8 minutes, shaling once. Serve warm.

2. Air Fried Green Tomatoes(1)

Servings: 4
Cooking Time: 20 Minutes
Ingredients:
- 2 medium green tomatoes
- ⅓ cup grated Parmesan cheese.
- ¼ cup blanched finely ground almond flour.
- 1 large egg.

Directions:
1. Slice tomatoes into ½-inch-thick slices. Take a medium bowl, whisk the egg. Take a large bowl, mix the almond flour and Parmesan.
2. Dip each tomato slice into the egg, then dredge in the almond flour mixture. Place the slices into the air fryer basket
3. Adjust the temperature to 400 Degrees F and set the timer for 7 minutes. Flip the slices halfway through the cooking time. Serve immediately
- **Nutrition Info:** Calories: 106; Protein: 6.2g; Fiber: 1.4g; Fat: 6.7g; Carbs: 5.9g

3. Garlic & Parmesan Bread Bites

Servings: 12
Cooking Time: 7 Minutes
Ingredients:
- 2 ciabatta loaves
- 1 stick butter at room temperature
- 4-6 crushed garlic cloves
- Chopped parsley
- 2 tablespoons finely grated parmesan

Directions:
1. Start by cutting bread in half and toasting it crust-side down for 2 minutes.
2. Mix the butter, garlic, and parsley together and spread over the bread.
3. Sprinkle parmesan over bread and toast in oven another 5 minutes.
- **Nutrition Info:** Calories: 191, Sodium: 382 mg, Dietary Fiber: 1.0 g, Total Fat: 9.4 g, Total Carbs: 21.7 g, Protein: 4.9 g.

4. Coriander Artichokes(1)

Servings: 4
Cooking Time: 20 Minutes
Ingredients:
- 12 oz. artichoke hearts
- 1 tbsp. lemon juice
- 1 tsp. coriander, ground
- ½ tsp. cumin seeds
- ½ tsp. olive oil
- Salt and black pepper to taste.

Directions:
1. In a pan that fits your air fryer, mix all the ingredients, toss, introduce the pan in the fryer and cook at 370°F for 15 minutes
2. Divide the mix between plates and serve as a side dish.
- **Nutrition Info:** Calories: 200; Fat: 7g; Fiber: 2g; Carbs: 5g; Protein: 8g

5. Shrimp With Spices

Servings: 3
Cooking Time: 15 Minutes
Ingredients:
- ½ pound shrimp, deveined
- ½ tsp Cajun seasoning
- Salt and black pepper to taste
- 1 tbsp olive oil
- ¼ tsp paprika

Directions:
1. Preheat Kalorik Maxx on Air Fry function to 390 F. In a bowl, mix paprika, salt, pepper, olive oil, and Cajun seasoning. Add in the shrimp and toss to coat. Transfer the prepared shrimp to the AirFryer basket and fit in the baking tray. Cook for 10-12 minutes, flipping halfway through.

6. Goat Cheese & Pancetta Bombs

Servings: 10
Cooking Time: 25 Minutes
Ingredients:
- 16 oz soft goat cheese
- 2 tbsp fresh rosemary, finely chopped
- 1 cup almonds, chopped into small pieces
- Salt and black pepper
- 15 dried plums, chopped
- 15 pancetta slices

Directions:
1. Line the Kalorik Maxx Air Fryer tray with parchment paper. In a bowl, add goat cheese, rosemary, almonds, salt, pepper, and plums; stir well. Roll into balls and wrap with pancetta slices. Arrange the bombs on the tray and cook for 10 minutes at 400 F. Let cool before serving.

7. Kale And Walnuts(1)

Servings: 4
Cooking Time: 8 Minutes
Ingredients:
- 3 garlic cloves
- 10 cups kale; roughly chopped.
- 1/3 cup parmesan; grated
- ½ cup almond milk
- ¼ cup walnuts; chopped.
- 1 tbsp. butter; melted
- ¼ tsp. nutmeg, ground
- Salt and black pepper to taste.

Directions:
1. In a pan that fits the air fryer, combine all the ingredients, toss, introduce the pan in the machine and cook at 360°F for 15 minutes
2. Divide between plates and serve.
- **Nutrition Info:** Calories: 160; Fat: 7g; Fiber: 2g; Carbs: 4g; Protein: 5g

8. Beef Enchilada Dip

Servings: 8
Cooking Time: 10 Minutes
Ingredients:
- 2 lbs. ground beef
- ½ onion, chopped fine
- 2 cloves garlic, chopped fine
- 2 cups enchilada sauce
- 2 cups Monterrey Jack cheese, grated
- 2 tbsp. sour cream

Directions:
1. Place rack in position
2. Heat a large skillet over med-high heat. Add beef and cook until it starts to brown. Drain off fat.
3. Stir in onion and garlic and cook until tender, about 3 minutes. Stir in enchilada sauce and transfer mixture to a small casserole dish and top with cheese.
4. Set oven to convection bake on 325°F for 10 minutes. After 5 minutes, add casserole to the oven and bake 3-5 minutes until cheese is melted and mixture is heated through.
5. Serve warm topped with sour cream.
- **Nutrition Info:** Calories 414, Total Fat 22g, Saturated Fat 10g, Total Carbs 15g, Net Carbs 11g, Protein 39g, Sugar 8g, Fiber 4g, Sodium 1155mg, Potassium 635mg, Phosphorus 385mg

9. Jicama Fries(3)

Servings: 4
Cooking Time: 20 Minutes
Ingredients:
- 1 small jicama; peeled.
- ¼ tsp. onion powder.
- ¾ tsp. chili powder
- ¼ tsp. ground black pepper
- ¼ tsp. garlic powder.

Directions:
1. Cut jicama into matchstick-sized pieces.
2. Place pieces into a small bowl and sprinkle with remaining ingredients. Place the fries into the air fryer basket
3. Adjust the temperature to 350 Degrees F and set the timer for 20 minutes. Toss the basket two or three times during cooking. Serve warm.

- **Nutrition Info:** Calories: 37; Protein: 8g; Fiber: 7g; Fat: 1g; Carbs: 7g

10. Parsley Mushroom Pilaf

Servings: 4
Cooking Time: 35 Minutes
Ingredients:
- 2 tbsp olive oil
- 2 cups heated vegetable stock
- 1 cups long-grain rice
- 1 onion, chopped
- 2 garlic cloves, minced
- 2 cups cremini mushrooms, chopped
- Salt and black pepper to taste
- 1 tbsp fresh parsley, chopped

Directions:
1. Preheat Kalorik Maxx on AirFry function to 400 F. Heat olive oil in a frying pan over medium heat. and sauté mushrooms, onion, and garlic for 5 minutes until tender. Stir in rice for 1-2 minutes.
2. Pour in the vegetable stock. Season with salt and pepper. Transfer to a baking dish and place in your Kalorik Maxx oven. Press Start and cook for 20 minutes. Serve sprinkled with chopped parsley.

11. Bok Choy And Butter Sauce(2)

Servings: 4
Cooking Time: 20 Minutes
Ingredients:
- 2 bok choy heads; trimmed and cut into strips
- 1 tbsp. butter; melted
- 2 tbsp. chicken stock
- 1 tsp. lemon juice
- 1 tbsp. olive oil
- A pinch of salt and black pepper

Directions:
1. In a pan that fits your air fryer, mix all the ingredients, toss, introduce the pan in the air fryer and cook at 380°F for 15 minutes.
2. Divide between plates and serve as a side dish
- **Nutrition Info:** Calories: 141; Fat: 3g; Fiber: 2g; Carbs: 4g; Protein: 3g

12. Cherry Farro

Servings: 6
Cooking Time: 40 Minutes
Ingredients:
- 1 teaspoon lemon juice Salt, to taste
- 1 tablespoon apple cider vinegar
- 1 cup whole grain faro
- 2 cups cherries, pitted and cut into halves
- 3 cups water
- ½ cup cherries, dried and chopped
- 1 tablespoon extra-virgin olive oil
- ¼ cup green onions, chopped
- 10 mint leaves, chopped

Directions:
1. Place the water in the Instant Pot, add the spelled rinse, stir, cover and cook in the Multigrain setting for 40 minutes.
2. Relieve the pressure, drain the spelled, transfer it to a bowl and mix with salt, oil, lemon juice, vinegar, dried cherries, fresh cherries, green onions and mint. Mix well, divide between plates and serve.
- **Nutrition Info:** Calories: 160, Fat: 1, Fiber: 2, Carbohydrate: 12, Proteins: 4

13. Baked Artichoke Hearts

Servings: 6
Cooking Time: 25 Minutes
Ingredients:
- 15 oz frozen artichoke hearts, defrosted
- 1 tbsp olive oil
- Pepper
- Salt

Directions:
1. Fit the Kalorik Maxx oven with the rack in position
2. Arrange artichoke hearts in baking pan and drizzle with olive oil. Season with pepper and salt.
3. Set to bake at 400 F for 30 minutes. After 5 minutes place the baking pan in the preheated oven.
4. Serve and enjoy.
- **Nutrition Info:** Calories 53 Fat 2.4 g Carbohydrates 7.5 g Sugar 0.7 g Protein 2.3 g Cholesterol 0 mg

14. Homemade Chicken Thighs

Servings: 4
Cooking Time: 30 Minutes
Ingredients:
- 1 pound chicken thighs
- ½ tsp salt
- ¼ tsp black pepper
- ¼ tsp garlic powder

Directions:
1. Season the thighs with salt, pepper, and garlic powder. Arrange them, skin side down on the frying basket. Select Bake function, adjust the temperature to 380 F, and press Start. Bake until golden brown, about 20 minutes. Serve warm.

15. Polenta Sticks

Servings: 4
Cooking Time: 6 Minutes
Ingredients:
- 1 tablespoon oil
- 2½ cups cooked polenta
- Salt, to taste
- ¼ cup Parmesan cheese

Directions:
1. Place the polenta in a lightly greased baking pan.
2. With a plastic wrap, cover and refrigerate for about 1 hour or until set.
3. Remove from the refrigerator and cut into desired sized slices.
4. Sprinkle with salt.
5. Press "Power Button" of Air Fry Oven and turn the dial to select the "Air Fry" mode.
6. Press the Time button and again turn the dial to set the cooking time to 6 minutes.
7. Now push the Temp button and rotate the dial to set the temperature at 350 degrees F.
8. Press "Start/Pause" button to start.
9. When the unit beeps to show that it is preheated, open the lid.
10. Arrange the pan over the "Wire Rack" and insert in the oven.
11. Top with cheese and serve.
- **Nutrition Info:** Calories 397 Total Fat 5.6g Saturated Fat 1.3 g Cholesterol 4mg Sodium 127 mg Total Carbs 76.2 g Fiber 2.5 g Sugar 1 g Protein 9.1 g

16. Healthy Asparagus Potatoes

Servings: 4
Cooking Time: 35 Minutes
Ingredients:
- 9 oz asparagus, cut into 2-inch pieces
- 2 lbs potatoes, cut into quarters
- 1/4 cup balsamic vinegar
- 2 tbsp olive oil

Directions:
1. Fit the Kalorik Maxx oven with the rack in position
2. In a large bowl, add potatoes, balsamic vinegar, olive oil, and salt and toss well.
3. Spread potatoes in baking pan.
4. Set to bake at 390 F for 25 minutes. After 5 minutes place the baking pan in the preheated oven.
5. Add asparagus and stir well and bake for 15 minutes more.
6. Season with pepper and salt.
7. Serve and enjoy.
- **Nutrition Info:** Calories 232 Fat 7.3 g Carbohydrates 38.3 g Sugar 3.9 g Protein 5.2 g Cholesterol 0 mg

17. Party Macaroni Quiche With Greek Yogurt

Servings: 4
Cooking Time: 30 Minutes
Ingredients:
- 8 tbsp leftover macaroni with cheese
- Extra cheese for serving
- Pastry as much needed for forming 4 shells
- Salt and black pepper to taste
- 1 tsp garlic puree
- 2 tbsp Greek yogurt
- 2 whole eggs
- 12 oz milk

Directions:
1. Preheat Kalorik Maxx on Air Fry function to 360 F. Roll the pastry to form 4 shells. Place them in the Air Fryer pan.
2. In a bowl, mix leftover macaroni with cheese, yogurt, eggs, milk, and garlic puree. Spoon this mixture into the pastry shells. Top with the cheese evenly. Cook for 20 minutes.

18. Baked Sweet Potatoes

Servings: 6
Cooking Time: 35 Minutes
Ingredients:
- 4 large sweet potatoes, peel and cut into cubes
- 8 sage leaves
- 1 tsp honey
- 2 tsp vinegar
- 1/2 tsp paprika
- 2 tbsp olive oil
- 1/2 tsp sea salt

Directions:
1. Fit the Kalorik Maxx oven with the rack in position
2. Add sweet potato, oil, sage, and salt in a baking dish and mix well.
3. Set to bake at 375 F for 40 minutes. After 5 minutes place the baking dish in the preheated oven.
4. Transfer roasted sweet potatoes into the large bowl and toss with honey, vinegar, and paprika.
5. Serve and enjoy.
- **Nutrition Info:** Calories 92 Fat 5.1 g Carbohydrates 12 g Sugar 1.2 g Protein 0.8 g Cholesterol 0 mg

19. Homemade Cod Fingers

Servings: 3
Cooking Time: 25 Minutes
Ingredients:
- 2 cups flour
- Salt and black pepper to taste
- 1 tsp seafood seasoning
- 2 whole eggs, beaten
- 1 cup cornmeal
- 1 pound cod fillets, cut into fingers
- 2 tbsp milk
- 2 eggs, beaten
- 1 cup breadcrumbs
- 1 lemon, cut into wedges

Directions:
1. Preheat Kalorik Maxx on Air Fryer function to 400 F. In a bowl, mix beaten eggs with milk. In a separate bowl, combine flour, cornmeal, and seafood seasoning. In another mixing bowl, mix spices with the eggs. In a third bowl, pour the breadcrumbs.
2. Dip cod fingers in the seasoned flour mixture, followed by a dip in the egg mixture, and finally coat with breadcrumbs. Place the fingers in your Air Fryer basket and fit in the baking tray. Cook for 10 minutes until golden brown. Serve with lemon wedges.

20. Potato Chips With Creamy Lemon Dip

Servings: 3
Cooking Time: 25 Minutes
Ingredients:
- 3 large potatoes
- 1 cup sour cream
- 2 scallions, white part minced
- 3 tbsp olive oil.
- ½ tsp lemon juice
- salt and black pepper

Directions:
1. Preheat Kalorik Maxx on AirFry function to 350 F. Cut the potatoes into thin slices; do not peel them. Brush them with olive oil and season with salt and pepper. Arrange on the frying basket.
2. Press Start on the oven and cook for 20-25 minutes. Season with salt and pepper. To prepare the dip, mix together the sour cream, olive oil, scallions, lemon juice, salt, and pepper.

21. Mashed Squash

Servings: 4
Cooking Time: 20 Minutes
Ingredients:
- 2 acorn squashes, cut into halves and seeded
- ½ cup water
- ¼ teaspoon baking soda
- 2 tablespoons butter
- Salt and ground black pepper, to taste
- ½ teaspoon fresh nutmeg, grated
- 2 tablespoons brown sugar

Directions:
1. Sprinkle the pumpkin halves with salt, pepper and baking soda and place them in the steam basket of the Instant Pot.

2. Add water to the Instant Pot, cover and cook for 20 minutes in manual configuration. Relieve the pressure, take the pumpkin and set it on a plate to cool. Scrape the flesh of the pumpkin and place it in a bowl.
3. Add salt, pepper, butter, sugar and nutmeg and mash with a potato masher. Mix well and serve.
- **Nutrition Info:** Calories: 140, Fat: 1, Fiber: 0.5, Carbohydrate: 10.5, Proteins: 1.7

22. Roasted Radishes With Brown Butter, Lemon, And Radish Tops

Servings: 4
Cooking Time: 20 Minutes
Ingredients:
- 2 bunches medium radishes
- 1-1/2 tablespoons olive oil
- Coarse kosher salt
- 2 tablespoons (1/4 stick) unsalted butter
- 1 teaspoon fresh lemon juice

Directions:
1. Start by preheating toaster oven to 450°F.
2. Cut tops off radishes (about 1/2-inch) and coarsely chop them and set aside.
3. Cut radishes down the middle lengthwise and place in a large bowl.
4. Add olive oil to the bowl and toss to coat. Place radishes flat side down and sprinkle with salt. Roast radishes in a pan for 20 minutes.
5. Toward the end of the roasting time, melt the butter in a small sauce pan until it browns and add lemon juice.
6. Transfer the radishes to a serving bowl; drizzle with butter, sprinkle with chopped radish tops, and serve.
- **Nutrition Info:** Calories: 96, Sodium: 42 mg, Dietary Fiber: 0 g, Total Fat: 11.0 g, Total Carbs: 0.1 g, Protein: 0.1 g.

23. Spinach And Artichokes Sauté

Servings: 4
Cooking Time: 20 Minutes
Ingredients:
- 10 oz. artichoke hearts; halved
- 2 cups baby spinach
- 3 garlic cloves
- ¼ cup veggie stock
- 2 tsp. lime juice
- Salt and black pepper to taste.

Directions:
1. In a pan that fits your air fryer, mix all the ingredients, toss, introduce in the fryer and cook at 370°F for 15 minutes
2. Divide between plates and serve as a side dish.
- **Nutrition Info:** Calories: 209; Fat: 6g; Fiber: 2g; Carbs: 4g; Protein: 8g

24. Sesame Garlic Chicken Wings

Servings: 4
Cooking Time: 55 Minutes
Ingredients:
- 1 pound chicken wings
- 1 cup soy sauce, divided
- ½ cup brown sugar
- ½ cup apple cider vinegar
- 2 tbsp fresh ginger, minced
- 2 tbsp fresh garlic, minced
- 1 tsp finely ground black pepper
- 2 tbsp cornstarch
- 2 tbsp cold water
- 1 tsp sesame seeds

Directions:
1. In a bowl, mix the chicken wings with a half cup of the soy sauce. Refrigerate for 20 minutes; drain and pat dry. Arrange the wings on the Air Fryer basket and fit in the baking tray. Cook for 20 minutes at 380 F on Air Fry function, turning once halfway through.
2. In a skillet over medium heat, stir sugar, remaining soy sauce, vinegar, ginger, garlic, and pepper. Cook until sauce has reduced slightly. Dissolve cornstarch in cold water and stir in the sauce; cook until it thickens, 2 minutes. Pour the sauce over wings and sprinkle with sesame seeds.

25. Winter Vegetables With Herbs

Servings: 2
Cooking Time: 20 Minutes
Ingredients:
- 1/2-pound broccoli florets

- 1 celery root, peeled and cut into 1-inch pieces
- 1 onion, cut into wedges
- 2 tablespoons unsalted butter, melted
- 1/2 cup chicken broth
- 1/4 cup tomato sauce
- 1 teaspoon parsley
- 1 teaspoon rosemary
- 1 teaspoon thyme

Directions:
1. Start by preheating your Air Fryer to 380 degrees F. Place all ingredients in a lightly greased casserole dish. Stir to combine well.
2. Bake in the preheated Air Fryer for 10 minutes. Gently stir the vegetables with a large spoon and cook for 5 minutes more.
3. Serve in individual bowls with a few drizzles of lemon juice.

- **Nutrition Info:** 141 Calories; 13g Fat; 1g Carbs; 5g Protein; 9g Sugars; 6g Fiber

26. Chili Lime Sweet Potatoes

Servings: 4
Cooking Time: 15 Minutes
Ingredients:
- 2 large sweet potatoes, peeled & cut into 1-inch pieces
- 1 tbsp chili powder
- 2 tbsp olive oil
- 2 tsp fresh lime juice
- 1 tsp cumin

Directions:
1. Fit the Kalorik Maxx oven with the rack in position 2.
2. In a mixing bowl, add sweet potatoes, lime juice, cumin, chili powder, and olive oil and toss well.
3. Transfer sweet potatoes in air fryer basket then place air fryer basket in baking pan.
4. Place a baking pan on the oven rack. Set to air fry at 380 F for 20 minutes.
5. Serve and enjoy.

- **Nutrition Info:** Calories 132 Fat 1.1 g Carbohydrates 17.1 g Sugar 0.8 g Protein 1.2 g Cholesterol 0 mg

27. Crispy Zucchini Sticks

Servings: 4
Cooking Time: 14 Minutes
Ingredients:
- 2 small zucchini, cut into 2-inch × ½-inch sticks
- 3 tablespoons chickpea flour
- 2 teaspoons arrowroot (or cornstarch)
- ½ teaspoon garlic granules
- ¼ teaspoon sea salt
- ⅛ teaspoon freshly ground black pepper
- 1 tablespoon water
- Cooking spray

Directions:
1. Combine the zucchini sticks with the chickpea flour, arrowroot, garlic granules, salt, and pepper in a medium bowl and toss to coat. Add the water and stir to mix well.
2. Spritz the air fryer basket with cooking spray and spread out the zucchini sticks in the pan. Mist the zucchini sticks with cooking spray.
3. Put the air fryer basket on the baking pan and slide into Rack Position 2, select Air Fry, set temperature to 392ºF (200ºC), and set time to 14 minutes.
4. Stir the sticks halfway through the cooking time.
5. When cooking is complete, the zucchini sticks should be crispy and nicely browned. Remove from the oven and serve warm.

28. Sweet Carrot Puree

Servings: 4
Cooking Time: 5 Minutes
Ingredients:
- Salt, to taste
- 1 cup water
- 1 teaspoon brown sugar
- 1½ pounds carrots, peeled and chopped
- 1 tablespoon butter, softened
- 1 tablespoon honey

Directions:
1. Place the carrots in the Instant Pot, add the water, cover and cook for 4 minutes in the Manual setting.
2. Release the pressure naturally, drain the carrots and place them in a bowl.

3. Mix with an immersion blender, add the butter, salt and honey. Mix again, add the sugar on top and serve.
- **Nutrition Info:** Calories: 50, Fat: 1, Fiber: 3, Carbohydrate: 11, Proteins: 1

29. Cheddar & Prosciutto Strips

Servings: 6
Cooking Time: 50 Minutes
Ingredients:
- 1 lb cheddar cheese
- 12 prosciutto slices
- 1 cup flour
- 2 eggs, beaten
- 4 tbsp olive oil
- 1 cup breadcrumbs

Directions:
1. Cut the cheese into 6 equal pieces. Wrap each piece with 2 prosciutto slices. Place them in the freezer just enough to set, about 5 minutes; note that they mustn't be frozen.
2. Preheat Kalorik Maxx on AirFry function to 390 F. Dip the Strips into flour first, then in eggs, and coat with breadcrumbs. Place in the frying basket and drizzle with olive oil. Press Start and cook for 10 minutes or until golden brown. Serve with tomato dip.

30. Parmesan Cauliflower

Servings: 5 Cups
Cooking Time: 15 Minutes
Ingredients:
- 8 cups small cauliflower florets (about 1¼ pounds / 567 g)
- 3 tablespoons olive oil
- 1 teaspoon garlic powder
- ½ teaspoon salt
- ½ teaspoon turmeric
- ¼ cup shredded Parmesan cheese

Directions:
1. In a bowl, combine the cauliflower florets, olive oil, garlic powder, salt, and turmeric and toss to coat. Transfer to the air fryer basket.
2. Put the air fryer basket on the baking pan and slide into Rack Position 2, select Air Fry, set temperature to 390ºF (199ºC), and set time to 15 minutes.
3. After 5 minutes, remove from the oven and stir the cauliflower florets. Return to the oven and continue cooking.
4. After 6 minutes, remove from the oven and stir the cauliflower. Return to the oven and continue cooking for 4 minutes. The cauliflower florets should be crisp-tender.
5. When cooking is complete, remove from the oven to a plate. Sprinkle with the shredded Parmesan cheese and toss well. Serve warm.

31. Kale And Walnuts(2)

Servings: 4
Cooking Time: 20 Minutes
Ingredients:
- 3 garlic cloves
- 10 cups kale; roughly chopped.
- 1/3 cup parmesan; grated
- ½ cup almond milk
- ¼ cup walnuts; chopped.
- 1 tbsp. butter; melted
- ¼ tsp. nutmeg, ground
- Salt and black pepper to taste.

Directions:
1. In a pan that fits the air fryer, combine all the ingredients, toss, introduce the pan in the machine and cook at 360°F for 15 minutes
2. Divide between plates and serve.
- **Nutrition Info:** Calories: 160; Fat: 7g; Fiber: 2g; Carbs: 4g; Protein: 5g

32. Cheesy Garlic Biscuits

Servings: 4
Cooking Time: 20 Minutes
Ingredients:
- 1 large egg.
- 1 scallion, sliced
- ¼ cup unsalted butter; melted and divided
- ½ cup shredded sharp Cheddar cheese.
- 1/3 cup coconut flour
- ½ tsp. baking powder.
- ½ tsp. garlic powder.

Directions:
1. Take a large bowl, mix coconut flour, baking powder and garlic powder.
2. Stir in egg, half of the melted butter, Cheddar cheese and scallions. Pour the

mixture into a 6-inch round baking pan. Place into the air fryer basket
3. Adjust the temperature to 320 Degrees F and set the timer for 12 minutes
4. To serve, remove from pan and allow to fully cool. Slice into four pieces and pour remaining melted butter over each.
- **Nutrition Info:** Calories: 218; Protein: 7.2g; Fiber: 3.4g; Fat: 16.9g; Carbs: 6.8g

33. Homemade Prosciutto Wrapped Cheese Sticks

Servings: 6
Cooking Time: 50 Minutes
Ingredients:
- 1 lb cheddar cheese
- 12 slices of prosciutto
- 1 cup flour
- 2 eggs, beaten
- 4 tbsp olive oil
- 1 cup breadcrumbs

Directions:
1. Cut the cheese into 6 equal sticks. Wrap each piece with 2 prosciutto slices. Place them in the freezer just enough to set. Preheat Kalorik Maxx on Air Fry function to 390 F. Dip the croquettes into flour first, then in eggs, and coat with breadcrumbs. Drizzle the basket with oil and fit in the baking tray. Cook for 10 minutes or until golden. Serve.

34. Rosemary Chickpeas

Servings: 4
Cooking Time: 20 Minutes
Ingredients:
- 2 (14.5-ounce) cans chickpeas, rinsed
- 2 tbsp olive oil
- 1 tsp dried rosemary
- ½ tsp dried thyme
- ¼ tsp dried sage
- ¼ tsp salt

Directions:
1. In a bowl, mix together chickpeas, oil, rosemary, thyme, sage, and salt. Transfer to a baking pan. Select Bake function, adjust the temperature to 380 F, and press Start. Cook for 15 minutes.

35. Bacon & Potato Salad With Mayonnaise

Servings: 6
Cooking Time: 10 Minutes
Ingredients:
- 4 lb boiled and cubed potatoes
- 15 bacon slices, chopped
- 2 cups shredded cheddar cheese
- 15 oz sour cream
- 2 tbsp mayonnaise
- 1 tsp salt
- 1 tsp pepper
- 1 tsp dried herbs, any

Directions:
1. Preheat Kalorik Maxx on Air Fry function to 350 F. Combine the potatoes, bacon, salt, pepper, and herbs in a large bowl. Transfer to the Kalorik Maxx baking pan. Cook for about 7 minutes. Remove and stir in sour cream and mayonnaise and serve.

36. Tasty Hassel Back Potatoes

Servings: 4
Cooking Time: 30 Minutes
Ingredients:
- 4 potatoes, peel & cut potato across the potato to make 1/8-inch slices
- 1/4 cup parmesan cheese, shredded
- 1 tbsp olive oil

Directions:
1. Fit the Kalorik Maxx oven with the rack in position 2.
2. Brush potatoes with olive oil.
3. Place potatoes in the air fryer basket then place an air fryer basket in the baking pan.
4. Place a baking pan on the oven rack. Set to air fry at 350 F for 30 minutes.
5. Sprinkle cheese on top of potatoes and serve.
- **Nutrition Info:** Calories 195 Fat 4.9 g Carbohydrates 33.7 g Sugar 2.5 g Protein 5.4 g Cholesterol 4 mg

37. Baked Broccoli

Servings: 6
Cooking Time: 20 Minutes
Ingredients:

- 4 cups broccoli florets
- 3 tbsp olive oil
- 1/2 tsp pepper
- 1/2 tsp garlic powder
- 1 tsp Italian seasoning
- 1 tsp salt

Directions:
1. Fit the Kalorik Maxx oven with the rack in position
2. Spread broccoli in baking pan and drizzle with oil and season with garlic powder, Italian seasoning, pepper, and salt.
3. Set to bake at 400 F for 25 minutes. After 5 minutes place the baking pan in the preheated oven.
4. Serve and enjoy.
- **Nutrition Info:** Calories 84 Fat 7.4 g Carbohydrates 4.4 g Sugar 1.2 g Protein 1.8 g Cholesterol 1 mg

38. Crispy Cauliflower Poppers

Servings: 4
Cooking Time: 20 Minutes
Ingredients:
- 1 egg white
- 1½ tablespoons ketchup
- 1 tablespoon hot sauce
- 1/3 cup panko breadcrumbs
- 2 cups cauliflower florets

Directions:
1. In a shallow bowl, mix together the egg white, ketchup and hot sauce.
2. In another bowl, place the breadcrumbs.
3. Dip the cauliflower florets in ketchup mixture and then coat with the breadcrumbs.
4. Press "Power Button" of Air Fry Oven and turn the dial to select the "Air Fry" mode.
5. Press the Time button and again turn the dial to set the cooking time to 20 minutes.
6. Now push the Temp button and rotate the dial to set the temperature at 320 degrees F.
7. Press "Start/Pause" button to start.
8. When the unit beeps to show that it is preheated, open the lid.
9. Arrange the cauliflower florets in "Air Fry Basket" and insert in the oven.
10. Toss the cauliflower florets once halfway through.
11. Serve warm.
- **Nutrition Info:** Calories 55 Total Fat 0.7 g Saturated Fat 0.3g Cholesterol 0 mg Sodium 181 mg Total Carbs 5.6 g Fiber 1.3 g Sugar 2.6 g Protein 2.3 g

39. Glazed Carrots

Servings: 4
Cooking Time: 6 Minutes
Ingredients:
- 1 pound baby carrots
- ½ cup water
- ½ cup honey
- 2 tablespoons butter
- 1 teaspoon dried thyme
- 1 teaspoon dried dill Salt, to taste

Directions:
1. Place the water in the Instant Pot, place the carrots in the steam basket, cover and cook for 3 minutes in the Manual setting.
2. Relieve the pressure, drain the carrots and place them in a bowl. Put the Instant Pot in the sauté mode, add the butter and melt. Add the dill, thyme, honey and salt and mix well.
3. Add the carrots, mix to coat, cook for 1 minute, transfer to the dishes and serve.
- **Nutrition Info:** Calories: 200, Fat: 11, Fiber: 4, Carbohydrate: 12, Proteins: 1.4

BREAKFAST RECIPES

40. Prosciutto & Mozzarella Crostini

Servings: 1
Cooking Time: 7 Minutes
Ingredients:
- ½ cup finely chopped tomatoes
- 3 oz chopped mozzarella
- 3 prosciutto slices, chopped
- 1 tbsp olive oil
- 1 tsp dried basil
- 6 small slices of French bread

Directions:
1. Preheat Kalorik Maxx on Toast function to 350 F. Place the bread slices in the toaster oven and toast for 5 minutes. Top the bread with tomatoes, prosciutto and mozzarella. Sprinkle the basil over the mozzarella. Drizzle with olive oil. Return to oven and cook for 1 more minute, enough to become melty and warm.

41. Egg Florentine With Spinach

Servings: 4
Cooking Time: 15 Minutes
Ingredients:
- 3 cups frozen spinach, thawed and drained
- 2 tablespoons heavy cream
- ¼ teaspoon kosher salt
- ⅛ teaspoon freshly ground black pepper
- 4 ounces (113 g) Ricotta cheese
- 2 garlic cloves, minced
- ½ cup panko bread crumbs
- 3 tablespoons grated Parmesan cheese
- 2 teaspoons unsalted butter, melted
- 4 large eggs

Directions:
1. In a medium bowl, whisk together the spinach, heavy cream, salt, pepper, Ricotta cheese and garlic.
2. In a small bowl, whisk together the bread crumbs, Parmesan cheese and butter. Set aside.
3. Spoon the spinach mixture into the baking pan and form four even circles.
4. Slide the baking pan into Rack Position 2, select Roast, set temperature to 375ºF (190ºC) and set time to 15 minutes.
5. After 8 minutes, remove the pan. The spinach should be bubbling. With the back of a large spoon, make indentations in the spinach for the eggs. Crack the eggs into the indentations and sprinkle the panko mixture over the surface of the eggs.
6. Return the pan to the oven and continue cooking.
7. When cooking is complete, remove the pan from the oven. Serve hot.

42. Eggplant Hoagies

Servings: 3 Hoagies
Cooking Time: 12 Minutes
Ingredients:
- 6 peeled eggplant slices (about ½ inch thick and 3 inches in diameter)
- ¼ cup jarred pizza sauce
- 6 tablespoons grated Parmesan cheese
- 3 Italian sub rolls, split open lengthwise, warmed
- Cooking spray

Directions:
1. Spritz the air fryer basket with cooking spray.
2. Arrange the eggplant slices in the pan and spritz with cooking spray.
3. Put the air fryer basket on the baking pan and slide into Rack Position 2, select Air Fry, set temperature to 350ºF (180ºC) and set time to 10 minutes.
4. Flip the slices halfway through the cooking time.
5. When cooked, the eggplant slices should be lightly wilted and tender.
6. Divide and spread the pizza sauce and cheese on top of the eggplant slice
7. Put the air fryer basket on the baking pan and slide into Rack Position 2, select Air Fry, set temperature to 375ºF (190ºC) and set time to 2 minutes.
8. When cooked, the cheese will be melted.
9. Assemble each sub roll with two slices of eggplant and serve immediately.

43. Ham And Cheese Toast

Servings: 1

Cooking Time: 6 Minutes
Ingredients:
- 1 slice bread
- 1 teaspoon butter, at room temperature
- 1 egg
- Salt and freshly ground black pepper, to taste
- 2 teaspoons diced ham
- 1 tablespoon grated Cheddar cheese

Directions:
1. On a clean work surface, use a 2½-inch biscuit cutter to make a hole in the center of the bread slice with about ½-inch of bread remaining.
2. Spread the butter on both sides of the bread slice. Crack the egg into the hole and season with salt and pepper to taste. Transfer the bread to the air fryer basket.
3. Put the air fryer basket on the baking pan and slide into Rack Position 2, select Air Fry, set temperature to 325ºF (163ºC), and set time to 6 minutes.
4. After 5 minutes, remove the pan from the oven. Scatter the cheese and diced ham on top and continue cooking for an additional 1 minute.
5. When cooking is complete, the egg should be set and the cheese should be melted. Remove the toast from the oven to a plate and let cool for 5 minutes before serving.

44. Stuffed Poblanos

Servings: 4
Cooking Time: 30 Minutes
Ingredients:
- ½ lb. spicy ground pork breakfast sausage
- 4 large poblano peppers
- 4 large eggs.
- ½ cup full-fat sour cream.
- 4 oz. full-fat cream cheese; softened.
- ¼ cup canned diced tomatoes and green chiles, drained
- 8 tbsp. shredded pepper jack cheese

Directions:
1. In a medium skillet over medium heat, crumble and brown the ground sausage until no pink remains. Remove sausage and drain the fat from the pan. Crack eggs into the pan, scramble and cook until no longer runny
2. Place cooked sausage in a large bowl and fold in cream cheese. Mix in diced tomatoes and chiles. Gently fold in eggs
3. Cut a 4"–5" slit in the top of each poblano, removing the seeds and white membrane with a small knife. Separate the filling into four and spoon carefully into each pepper. Top each with 2 tbsp. pepper jack cheese
4. Place each pepper into the air fryer basket. Adjust the temperature to 350 Degrees F and set the timer for 15 minutes.
5. Peppers will be soft, and cheese will be browned when ready. Serve immediately with sour cream on top.
- **Nutrition Info:** Calories: 489; Protein: 22.8g; Fiber: 3.8g; Fat: 35.6g; Carbs: 12.6g

45. Healthy Baked Oatmeal

Servings: 6
Cooking Time: 20 Minutes
Ingredients:
- 1 egg
- 1/3 cup dried cranberries
- 1 tsp vanilla
- 1 1/2 tsp cinnamon
- 2 tbsp butter, melted
- 1/2 cup applesauce
- 1 1/2 cups milk
- 1 tsp baking powder
- 1/3 cup light brown sugar
- 2 cups old fashioned oats
- 1/4 tsp salt

Directions:
1. Fit the Kalorik Maxx oven with the rack in position
2. Grease 8*8-inch baking dish and set aside.
3. In a bowl, mix egg, vanilla, butter, applesauce, baking powder, cinnamon, brown sugar, oats, and salt.
4. Add milk and stir well.
5. Add cranberries and fold well.
6. Pour mixture into the prepared baking dish.
7. Set to bake at 350 F for 25 minutes. After 5 minutes place the baking dish in the preheated oven.
8. Serve and enjoy.

- **Nutrition Info:** Calories 330 Fat 9.3 g Carbohydrates 50.6 g Sugar 14.4 g Protein 9.7 g Cholesterol 42 mg

46. Savory Cheddar & Cauliflower Tater Tots

Servings: 4
Cooking Time: 35 Minutes
Ingredients:
- 2 lb cauliflower florets, steamed
- 5 oz cheddar cheese, shredded
- 1 onion, diced
- 1 cup breadcrumbs
- 1 egg, beaten
- 1 tsp fresh parsley, chopped
- 1 tsp fresh oregano, chopped
- 1 tsp fresh chives, chopped
- 1 tsp garlic powder
- Salt and black pepper to taste

Directions:
1. Mash the cauliflower and place it in a large bowl. Add in the onion, parsley, oregano, chives, garlic powder, salt, pepper, and cheddar cheese. Mix with your hands until thoroughly combined and form 12 balls out of the mixture.
2. Line a baking sheet with parchment paper. Dip half of the tater tots into the egg and then coat with breadcrumbs. Arrange them on the AirFryer Basket and spray with cooking spray.
3. Fit in the baking sheet and cook in the fryer oven at 390 minutes for 10-12 minutes on Air Fry function. Serve.

47. Raspberries Maple Pancakes

Servings: 4
Cooking Time: 15 Minutes
Ingredients:
- 2 cups all-purpose flour
- 1 cup milk
- 3 eggs, beaten
- 1 tsp baking powder
- 1 cup brown sugar
- 1 ½ tsp vanilla extract
- ½ cup frozen raspberries, thawed
- 2 tbsp maple syrup
- A pinch of salt

Directions:
1. Preheat Kalorik Maxx on Bake function to 400 F. In a bowl, mix the flour, baking powder, salt, milk, eggs, vanilla extract, and sugar until smooth. Stir in the raspberries. Do it gently to avoid coloring the batter.
2. Grease a pie pan with cooking spray. Drop the batter onto the pan. Make sure to leave some space between the pancakes. Cook for 10-15 minutes. Drizzle with maple syrup and serve.

48. Mozzarella Endives And Tomato Salad

Servings: 4
Cooking Time: 20 Minutes
Ingredients:
- 2 endives, shredded
- ½ pound cherry tomatoes, halved
- 1 tablespoon olive oil
- 4 eggs, whisked
- Salt and black pepper to the taste
- 1 teaspoon sweet paprika
- ½ cup mozzarella, shredded

Directions:
1. Preheat the air fryer with the oil at 350 degrees F, add the tomatoes, endives and the other ingredients except the mozzarella and toss.
2. Sprinkle the mozzarella on top, cook for 20 minutes, divide into bowls and serve for breakfast.
- **Nutrition Info:** calories 229, fat 13, fiber 3, carbs 4, protein 7

49. Quick Mac & Cheese

Servings: 2
Cooking Time: 15 Minutes
Ingredients:
- 1 cup macaroni, cooked
- 1 cup cheddar cheese, grated
- ½ cup warm milk
- 1 tbsp Parmesan cheese, grated
- Salt and black pepper to taste

Directions:
1. Preheat Kalorik Maxx on AirFry function to 350 F. Add the macaroni to an ovenproof baking dish. Stir in the cheddar cheese and milk. Season with salt and pepper. Place the

dish in the Kalorik Maxx oven and press Start. Cook for 10 minutes. Sprinkle with Parmesan cheese and serve.

50. Healthy Tofu Omelet

Servings: 2
Cooking Time: 29 Minutes
Ingredients:
- ¼ of onion, chopped
- 12-ounce silken tofu, pressed and sliced
- 3 eggs, beaten
- 1 tablespoon chives, chopped
- 1 garlic clove, minced
- 2 teaspoons olive oil
- Salt and black pepper, to taste

Directions:
1. Preheat the Air fryer to 355 ºF and grease an Air fryer pan with olive oil.
2. Add onion and garlic to the greased pan and cook for about 4 minutes.
3. Add tofu, mushrooms and chives and season with salt and black pepper.
4. Beat the eggs and pour over the tofu mixture.
5. Cook for about 25 minutes, poking the eggs twice in between
6. Dish out and serve warm.
- **Nutrition Info:** Calories: 248 Cal Total Fat: 15.9 g Saturated Fat: 0 g Cholesterol: 0 mg Sodium: 155 mg Total Carbs: 6.5 g Fiber: 0 g Sugar: 3.3 g Protein: 20.4 g

51. Chicken & Zucchini Omelet

Servings: 6
Cooking Time: 35 Minutes
Ingredients:
- 8 eggs
- ½ cup milk
- Salt and ground black pepper, as required
- 1 cup cooked chicken, chopped
- 1 cup Cheddar cheese, shredded
- ½ cup fresh chives, chopped
- ¾ cup zucchini, chopped

Directions:
1. In a bowl, add the eggs, milk, salt and black pepper and beat well.
2. Add the remaining ingredients and stir to combine.
3. Place the mixture into a greased baking pan.
4. Press "Power Button" of Air Fry Oven and turn the dial to select the "Air Bake" mode.
5. Press the Time button and again turn the dial to set the cooking time to 35 minutes.
6. Now push the Temp button and rotate the dial to set the temperature at 315 degrees F.
7. Press "Start/Pause" button to start.
8. When the unit beeps to show that it is preheated, open the lid.
9. Arrange pan over the "Wire Rack" and insert in the oven.
10. Cut into equal-sized wedges and serve hot.
- **Nutrition Info:** Calories 209 Total Fat 13.3 g Saturated Fat 6.3 g Cholesterol 258 mg Sodium 252 mg Total Carbs 2.3 g Fiber 0.3 g Sugar 1.8 g Protein 9.8 g

52. Easy Cheesy Breakfast Casserole

Servings: 8
Cooking Time: 30 Minutes
Ingredients:
- 6 eggs, lightly beaten
- 8 oz can crescent rolls
- 2 cups cheddar cheese, shredded
- 1 lb breakfast sausage, cooked

Directions:
1. Fit the Kalorik Maxx oven with the rack in position
2. Spray a 9*13-inch baking dish with cooking spray and set aside.
3. Spread crescent rolls in the bottom of the prepared baking dish and top with sausage, egg, and cheese.
4. Set to bake at 350 F for 35 minutes. After 5 minutes place the baking dish in the preheated oven.
5. Serve and enjoy.
- **Nutrition Info:** Calories 465 Fat 34.6 g Carbohydrates 11.8 g Sugar 2.4 g Protein 24.2 g Cholesterol 200 mg

53. Crustless Broccoli Quiche

Servings: 4
Cooking Time: 10 Minutes
Ingredients:
- 1 cup broccoli florets
- ¾ cup chopped roasted red peppers

- 1¼ cups grated Fontina cheese
- 6 eggs
- ¾ cup heavy cream
- ½ teaspoon salt
- Freshly ground black pepper, to taste
- Cooking spray

Directions:
1. Spritz the baking pan with cooking spray
2. Add the broccoli florets and roasted red peppers to the pan and scatter the grated Fontina cheese on top.
3. In a bowl, beat together the eggs and heavy cream. Sprinkle with salt and pepper. Pour the egg mixture over the top of the cheese. Wrap the pan in foil.
4. Put the air fryer basket on the baking pan and slide into Rack Position 2, select Air Fry, set temperature to 325ºF (163ºC) and set time to 10 minutes.
5. After 8 minutes, remove the pan from the oven. Remove the foil. Return to the oven and continue to cook for another 2 minutes.
6. When cooked, the quiche should be golden brown.
7. Rest for 5 minutes before cutting into wedges and serve warm.

54. Whole Wheat Carrot Bread

Servings: 10
Cooking Time: 50 Minutes
Ingredients:
- 1 egg
- 3/4 cup whole wheat flour
- 1 cup carrots, shredded
- 3/4 tsp vanilla
- 3/4 cup all-purpose flour
- 1/2 cup brown sugar
- 1 tsp baking powder
- 1/2 tsp nutmeg
- 1 1/2 tsp cinnamon
- 3/4 cup yogurt
- 3 tbsp vegetable oil
- 1 tsp baking soda

Directions:
1. Fit the Kalorik Maxx oven with the rack in position
2. In a large bowl, mix all dry ingredients and set aside.
3. In a separate bowl, whisk the egg with vanilla, sugar, yogurt, and oil.
4. Add carrots and fold well.
5. Add dry ingredient mixture and stir until just combined.
6. Pour mixture into the 9*5-inch greased loaf pan.
7. Set to bake at 350 F for 55 minutes, after 5 minutes, place the loaf pan in the oven.
8. Slice and serve.
- **Nutrition Info:** Calories 159 Fat 5 g Carbohydrates 24.4 g Sugar 9 g Protein 3.7 g Cholesterol 17 mg

55. Parmesan Asparagus

Servings: 4
Cooking Time: 20 Minutes
Ingredients:
- 1 lb asparagus spears
- ¼ cup flour
- 1 cup breadcrumbs
- ½ cup Parmesan cheese, grated
- 2 eggs, beaten
- Salt and black pepper to taste

Directions:
1. Preheat Kalorik Maxx on AirFry function to 370 F. Combine breadcrumbs, Parmesan cheese, salt, and pepper in a bowl. Line a baking sheet with parchment paper.
2. Dip the spears into the flour first, then into the eggs, and finally coat with the crumb mixture. Arrange them on a baking tray and press Start. Bake for 8-10 minutes. Serve warm.

56. Pumpkin And Yogurt Bread

Servings: 4
Cooking Time: 15 Minutes
Ingredients:
- 2 large eggs
- 8 tablespoons pumpkin puree
- 6 tablespoons banana flour
- 4 tablespoons plain Greek yogurt
- 6 tablespoons oats
- 4 tablespoons honey
- 2 tablespoons vanilla essence
- Pinch of ground nutmeg

Directions:

1. Preheat the Air fryer to 360 ºF and grease a loaf pan.
2. Mix together all the ingredients except oats in a bowl and beat with the hand mixer until smooth.
3. Add oats and mix until well combined.
4. Transfer the mixture into the prepared loaf pan and place in the Air fryer.
5. Cook for about 15 minutes and remove from the Air fryer.
6. Place onto a wire rack to cool and cut the bread into desired size slices to serve.
- **Nutrition Info:** Calories: 212 Cal Total Fat: 3.4 g Saturated Fat: 0 g Cholesterol: 0 mg Sodium: 49 mg Total Carbs: 36 g Fiber: 0 g Sugar: 20.5 g Protein: 6.6 g

57. Delicious Baked Omelet

Servings: 6
Cooking Time: 25 Minutes
Ingredients:
- 8 eggs
- 1/2 cup green bell pepper
- 1/2 cup onion, diced
- 1 cup ham, chopped & cooked
- 1 cup cheddar cheese, shredded
- 1/2 cup half and half
- Pepper
- Salt

Directions:
1. Fit the Kalorik Maxx oven with the rack in position
2. Spray 9*9-inch baking pan with cooking spray and set aside.
3. In a bowl, whisk eggs with half and half, pepper, and salt.
4. Add green bell pepper, onion, ham, and cheddar cheese and stir well.
5. Pour egg mixture into the prepared baking pan.
6. Set to bake at 400 F for 30 minutes. After 5 minutes place the baking pan in the preheated oven.
7. Serve and enjoy.
- **Nutrition Info:** Calories 230 Fat 16.4 g Carbohydrates 4.1 g Sugar 1.5 g Protein 16.6 g Cholesterol 258 mg

58. Banana & Peanut Butter Cake

Servings: 4
Cooking Time: 30 Minutes
Ingredients:
- 1 cup flour
- ¼ tsp baking soda
- 1 tsp baking powder
- ⅓ cup sugar
- 2 mashed bananas
- ¼ cup vegetable oil
- 1 egg, beaten
- 1 tsp vanilla extract
- ¾ cup chopped walnuts
- ¼ tsp salt
- 2 tbsp peanut butter
- 2 tbsp sour cream

Directions:
1. Preheat Kalorik Maxx on Bake function to 350 F. Spray a 9-inch baking pan with cooking spray or grease with butter. Combine the flour, salt, baking powder, and baking soda in a bowl.
2. In another bowl, combine bananas, oil, egg, peanut butter, vanilla, sugar, and sour cream. Combine both mixtures gently. Stir in the chopped walnuts. Pour the batter into the pan. Cook for 20 minutes. Let cool completely and serve sliced.

59. Spinach Zucchini Egg Muffins

Servings: 12
Cooking Time: 20 Minutes
Ingredients:
- 8 eggs
- 1 cup baby spinach, chopped
- 1 red bell pepper, diced
- 1/4 cup green onion, chopped
- 12 bacon slices, cooked and crumbled
- 2 small zucchini, sliced
- 1/4 cup almond milk
- 2 tbsp parsley, chopped
- 1 tbsp olive oil
- Pepper
- Salt

Directions:
1. Fit the Kalorik Maxx oven with the rack in position

2. Spray 12-cups muffin tin with cooking spray and set aside.
3. Heat olive oil in a pan over medium heat.
4. Add parsley, spinach, green onion, red bell pepper to the pan and sauté until spinach is wilted.
5. In a bowl, whisk eggs with almond milk, pepper, and salt.
6. Add sautéed vegetables, bacon, and zucchini to the egg mixture and stir well.
7. Pour egg mixture into the greased muffin tin.
8. Set to bake at 350 F for 25 minutes, after 5 minutes, place muffin tin in the oven.
9. Serve and enjoy.
- **Nutrition Info:** Calories 174 Fat 13.3 g Carbohydrates 2.5 g Sugar 1.3 g Protein 11.3 g Cholesterol 130 mg

60. Asparagus And Cheese Strata

Servings: 4
Cooking Time: 17 Minutes
Ingredients:
- 6 asparagus spears, cut into 2-inch pieces
- 1 tablespoon water
- 2 slices whole-wheat bread, cut into ½-inch cubes
- 4 eggs
- 3 tablespoons whole milk
- 2 tablespoons chopped flat-leaf parsley
- ½ cup grated Havarti or Swiss cheese
- Pinch salt
- Freshly ground black pepper, to taste
- Cooking spray

Directions:
1. Add the asparagus spears and 1 tablespoon of water in the baking pan.
2. Slide the baking pan into Rack Position 1, select Convection Bake, set temperature to 330ºF (166ºC) and set time to 4 minutes.
3. When cooking is complete, the asparagus spears will be crisp-tender.
4. Remove the asparagus from the pan and drain on paper towels.
5. Spritz the pan with cooking spray. Place the bread and asparagus in the pan.
6. Whisk together the eggs and milk in a medium mixing bowl until creamy. Fold in the parsley, cheese, salt, and pepper and stir to combine. Pour this mixture into the baking pan.
7. Select Bake and set time to 13 minutes. Put the pan back to the oven. When done, the eggs will be set and the top will be lightly browned.
8. Let cool for 5 minutes before slicing and serving.

61. Sweet Breakfast Casserole

Servings: 4
Cooking Time: 30 Minutes
Ingredients:
- 3 tablespoons brown sugar
- 4 tablespoons margarine
- 2 tablespoons white sugar
- 1/2 tsp. cinnamon powder
- 1/2 cup flour
- For the casserole:
- 2 eggs
- 2 tablespoons white sugar
- 2 and 1/2 cups white flour
- 1 tsp. baking soda
- 1 tsp. baking powder
- 2 eggs
- 1/2 cup milk
- 2 cups margarine milk
- 4 tablespoons margarine
- Zest from 1 lemon, grated
- 1 and 2/3 cup blueberries

Directions:
1. In a bowl, mix eggs with 2 tablespoons white sugar, 2 and 1/2 cups white flour, baking powder, baking soda, 2 eggs, milk, margarine milk, 4 tablespoons margarine, lemon zest and blueberries, stir and pour into a pan that fits your air fryer.
2. In another bowls, mix 3 tablespoons brown sugar with 2 tablespoons white sugar, 4 tablespoons margarine, 1/2 cup flour and cinnamon, stir until you obtain a crumble and spread over blueberries mix.
3. Place in preheated air fryer and bake at 300 °F for 30 minutes.
4. Divide among plates and serve for breakfast.

- **Nutrition Info:** Calories 101 Fat 9.4 g Carbohydrates 0.3 g Sugar 0.2 g Protein 7 g Cholesterol 21 mg

62. Banana Oat Muffins

Servings: 6
Cooking Time: 25 Minutes
Ingredients:
- 1 egg
- 2 tbsp butter, melted
- 1/2 tsp cinnamon
- 1 tsp vanilla
- 2 tbsp yogurt
- 1 1/2 cup oats
- 1 tsp baking powder
- 2 ripe bananas, mashed

Directions:
1. Fit the Kalorik Maxx oven with the rack in position
2. Line the muffin tray with cupcake liners and set aside.
3. In a bowl, whisk the egg with banana, yogurt, vanilla, cinnamon, baking powder, and butter.
4. Add oats and mix well.
5. Pour mixture into the prepared muffin tray.
6. Set to bake at 350 F for 30 minutes. After 5 minutes place the muffin tray in the preheated oven.
7. Serve and enjoy.
- **Nutrition Info:** Calories 164 Fat 6.1 g Carbohydrates 23.9 g Sugar 5.5 g Protein 4.4 g Cholesterol 38 mg

63. Bacon Bread Egg Casserole

Servings: 4
Cooking Time: 20 Minutes
Ingredients:
- 6 eggs
- 1 cup cheddar cheese, shredded
- 1/2 tsp garlic, minced
- 3 tbsp milk
- 2 tbsp green onion, chopped
- 1/3 bell pepper, diced
- 2 bread slices, cubed
- 5 bacon slices, diced
- Pepper
- Salt

Directions:
1. Fit the Kalorik Maxx oven with the rack in position
2. Add all ingredients into the large bowl and stir until well combined.
3. Pour into the greased baking dish.
4. Set to bake at 350 F for 25 minutes. After 5 minutes place the baking dish in the preheated oven.
5. Serve and enjoy.
- **Nutrition Info:** Calories 231 Fat 26.3 g Carbohydrates 5.2 g Sugar 1.9 g Protein 25 g Cholesterol 302 mg

64. Vanilla Granola

Servings: 4
Cooking Time: 40 Minutes
Ingredients:
- 1 cup rolled oats
- 3 tablespoons maple syrup
- 1 tablespoon sunflower oil
- 1 tablespoon coconut sugar
- ¼ teaspoon vanilla
- ¼ teaspoon cinnamon
- ¼ teaspoon sea salt

Directions:
1. Mix together the oats, maple syrup, sunflower oil, coconut sugar, vanilla, cinnamon, and sea salt in a medium bowl and stir to combine. Transfer the mixture to the baking pan.
2. Slide the baking pan into Rack Position 1, select Convection Bake, set temperature to 248ºF (120ºC) and set time to 40 minutes.
3. Stir the granola four times during cooking.
4. When cooking is complete, the granola will be mostly dry and lightly browned.
5. Let the granola stand for 5 to 10 minutes before serving.

65. Chicken Breakfast Sausages

Servings: 8 Patties
Cooking Time: 10 Minutes
Ingredients:
- 1 Granny Smith apple, peeled and finely chopped
- 2 tablespoons apple juice
- 2 garlic cloves, minced

- 1 egg white
- ⅓ cup minced onion
- 3 tablespoons ground almonds
- ⅛ teaspoon freshly ground black pepper
- 1 pound (454 g) ground chicken breast

Directions:
1. Combine all the ingredients except the chicken in a medium mixing bowl and stir well.
2. Add the chicken breast to the apple mixture and mix with your hands until well incorporated.
3. Divide the mixture into 8 equal portions and shape into patties. Arrange the patties in the air fryer basket.
4. Put the air fryer basket on the baking pan and slide into Rack Position 2, select Air Fry, set temperature to 330ºF (166ºC) and set time to 10 minutes.
5. When done, a meat thermometer inserted in the center of the chicken should reach at least 165ºF (74ºC).
6. Remove from the oven to a plate. Let the chicken cool for 5 minutes and serve warm.

66. Baked Peanut Butter Oatmeal

Servings: 4
Cooking Time: 35 Minutes
Ingredients:
- 2 cups old fashioned oats
- 2 tsp vanilla
- 1/4 cup maple syrup
- 1/2 cup peanut butter
- 1 3/4 cup almond milk
- 1/4 tsp salt

Directions:
1. Fit the Kalorik Maxx oven with the rack in position
2. In a mixing bowl, whisk together almond milk, vanilla, maple syrup, peanut butter, and salt.
3. Add oats and stir to mix.
4. Pour oats mixture into the greased baking dish.
5. Set to bake at 375 F for 40 minutes, after 5 minutes, place the baking dish in the oven.
6. Serve and enjoy.

- **Nutrition Info:** Calories 800 Fat 46.5 g Carbohydrates 79.3 g Sugar 20.6 g Protein 20.5 g Cholesterol 0 mg

67. Potato Egg Casserole

Servings: 6
Cooking Time: 35 Minutes
Ingredients:
- 5 eggs
- 2 medium potatoes, cut into 1/2-inch cubes
- 1 green bell pepper, diced
- 1 small onion, chopped
- 1 tbsp olive oil
- 1/2 cup cheddar cheese, shredded
- 3/4 tsp pepper
- 3/4 tsp salt

Directions:
1. Fit the Kalorik Maxx oven with the rack in position
2. Spray 9*9-inch casserole dish with cooking spray and set aside.
3. Heat oil in a pan over medium heat.
4. Add onion and sauté for 1 minute. Add potatoes, bell peppers, 1/2 tsp pepper, and 1/2 tsp salt and sauté for 4 minutes.
5. Transfer sautéed vegetables to the prepared casserole dish and spread evenly.
6. In a bowl, whisk eggs with remaining pepper and salt.
7. Pour egg mixture over sautéed vegetables in a casserole dish. Sprinkle cheese on top.
8. Set to bake at 350 F for 40 minutes. After 5 minutes place the casserole dish in the preheated oven.
9. Serve and enjoy.
- **Nutrition Info:** Calories 171 Fat 9.2 g Carbohydrates 14.3 g Sugar 2.6 g Protein 8.5 g Cholesterol 146 mg

68. Smoked Sausage Breakfast Mix

Servings: 4
Cooking Time: 30 Minutes
Ingredients:
- 1 and 1/2 pounds smoked sausage, diced and browned
- A pinch of salt and black pepper
- 1 and 1/2 cups grits
- 4 and 1/2 cups water

- 16 ounces cheddar cheese, shredded
- 1 cup milk
- ¼ tsp. garlic powder
- 1 and 1/2 tsp.s thyme, diced
- Cooking spray
- 4 eggs, whisked

Directions:
1. Put the water in a pot, bring to a boil over medium heat, add grits, stir, cover, cook for 5 minutes and take off heat.
2. Add cheese, stir until it melts and mix with milk, thyme, salt, pepper, garlic powder and eggs and whisk really well.
3. Heat up your air fryer at 300 °F, grease with cooking spray and add browned sausage.
4. Add grits mix, spread and cook for 25 minutes.
5. Divide among plates and serve for breakfast.
- **Nutrition Info:** Calories 113 Fat 8.2 g Carbohydrates 0.3 g Protein 5.4 g

69. Spinach & Kale Balsamic Chicken

Servings: 1
Cooking Time: 20 Minutes
Ingredients:
- ½ cup baby spinach leaves
- ½ cup shredded romaine
- 3 large kale leaves, chopped
- 4 oz chicken breasts, cut into cubes
- 3 tbsp olive oil, divided
- 1 tsp balsamic vinegar
- 1 garlic clove, minced
- Salt and black pepper to taste

Directions:
1. Place the chicken, 1 tbsp of olive oil, and garlic in a bowl. Season with salt and pepper and toss to combine. Put on a lined Air Fryer pan and cook for 14 minutes at 390 F on Bake function.
2. Place the greens in a large bowl. Add the remaining olive oil and balsamic vinegar. Season with salt and pepper and toss to combine. Top with the chicken and serve.

70. Beans And Pork Mix

Servings: 4
Cooking Time: 20 Minutes
Ingredients:

- 1-pound pork stew meat, ground
- 1 red onion, chopped
- 1 tablespoon olive oil
- 1 cup canned kidney beans, drained and rinsed
- 1 teaspoon chili powder
- Salt and black pepper to the taste
- ¼ teaspoon cumin, ground

Directions:
1. Heat up your air fryer at 360 degrees F, add the meat and the onion and cook for 5 minutes.
2. Add the beans and the rest of the ingredients, toss and cook for 15 minutes more.
3. Divide everything into bowls and serve for breakfast.
- **Nutrition Info:** calories 203, fat 4, fiber 6, carbs 12, protein 4

71. Oats, Chocolate Chip, Pecan Cookies

Servings:x
Cooking Time:x
Ingredients:
- ½ cup (115g) butter, softened
- ½ cup (100g) sugar
- 1 cup (170g) chocolate chips
- ½ cup (60g) pecan halves, chopped
- ½ cup (100g) firmly packed brown sugar
- 1 teaspoon vanilla extract
- 1 large egg
- 1L cup (160g) all-purpose flour
- 2 teaspoons baking powder
- ½ teaspoon kosher salt
- ¼ cup (20g) rolled oats

Directions:
1. Line 2 baking pans with parchment paper.
2. Assemble Kalorik Maxx bench mixer with beater attachment. Place butter, sugar, brown sugar and vanilla in the mixing bowl. Mix on medium speed for 2 minutes until pale and creamy.
3. Add egg and beat until just combined. Sift flour, baking powder and salt, then add to egg mixture on low speed, mixing until just combined.
4. Add chocolate chips, pecans and oats and mix on low speed until just combined.

5. Roll heaping tablespoons of dough into balls and place 6 balls, 2 inches (4cm) apart, on each prepared pan.
6. Insert wire racks in rack positions 3 and Select COOKIES/315°F (155°C)/SUPER CONVECTION/12 minutes. Press START to preheat oven.
7. Bake cookies for 12 minutes, rotating halfway through baking (change top to bottom and front to back).
8. Let cool on baking pans for 5 minutes then transfer to a wire rack to cool completely. 9. Repeat with remaining dough.

72. Egg And Avocado Burrito

Servings:4
Cooking Time: 4 Minutes
Ingredients:
- 4 low-sodium whole-wheat flour tortillas
- Filling:
- 1 hard-boiled egg, chopped
- 2 hard-boiled egg whites, chopped
- 1 ripe avocado, peeled, pitted, and chopped
- 1 red bell pepper, chopped
- 1 (1.2-ounce / 34-g) slice low-sodium, low-fat American cheese, torn into pieces
- 3 tablespoons low-sodium salsa, plus additional for serving (optional)
- Special Equipment:
- 4 toothpicks (optional), soaked in water for at least 30 minutes

Directions:
1. Make the filling: Combine the egg, egg whites, avocado, red bell pepper, cheese, and salsa in a medium bowl and stir until blended.
2. Assemble the burritos: Arrange the tortillas on a clean work surface and place ¼ of the prepared filling in the middle of each tortilla, leaving about 1½-inch on each end unfilled. Fold in the opposite sides of each tortilla and roll up. Secure with toothpicks through the center, if needed.
3. Transfer the burritos to the air fryer basket.
4. Put the air fryer basket on the baking pan and slide into Rack Position 2, select Air Fry, set temperature to 390ºF (199ºC) and set time to 4 minutes.
5. When cooking is complete, the burritos should be crisp and golden brown.
6. Allow to cool for 5 minutes and serve with salsa, if desired.

73. Avocado Oil Gluten Free Banana Bread Recipe

Servings:x
Cooking Time:x
Ingredients:
- 1/2 cup Granulated Sugar
- 1 cup Mashed Banana
- 1/2 cup Light Brown Sugar
- 1/3 cup Avocado Oil, (or canola oil)
- 2 cups All-Purpose Gluten Free Flour, (see notes)
- 3/4 teaspoon Xanthan Gum, (omit if your flour blend contains it)
- 1 teaspoon Baking Powder
- 1/2 teaspoon Baking Soda
- 1/2 teaspoon Fine Sea Salt
- 2 large Eggs, room temperature
- 2/3 cup Milk, (dairy free or regular milk), room temperature
- 1 teaspoon Pure Vanilla Extract

Directions:
1. Preheat oven to 350°F and spray a 9x9 inch square pan with non-stick spray and line with parchment paper.
2. In a large bowl, whisk together the flour, xanthan gum, baking powder, baking soda, salt, and granulated sugar.
3. In a separate bowl, whisk together the mashed banana, brown sugar, oil, eggs, milk, and vanilla extract. Pour the wet ingredients into the dry ingredients and stir to combine.
4. Pour the batter into the prepared pan and bake at 350°F for 25-30 minutes or until a toothpick or cake tester comes out clean or with a few moist crumbs attached. Cooking time will vary depending on your oven - mine took 29 minutes.
5. Cool the bread in the pan on a cooling rack. Cut into 16 pieces and serve slightly warm or room temperature.
6. To store, wrap tightly in foil or store slices in an air-tight container. It will stay fresh up

to 3 days. This bread also freezes well. To freeze, slice into individual pieces and freeze in a freezer bag.

74. Smart Oven Baked Oatmeal Recipe

Servings: x
Cooking Time: x
Ingredients:
- 1 small Ripe Banana, (6 inches long, abut 1/4 cup mashed)
- 1 tablespoon Flax Meal
- 1/2 cup Non-Dairy Milk, plus 2 tablespoons (like Almond Milk or Soy Milk)
- 1 cup Old Fashioned Rolled Oats
- 2 teaspoons Pure Maple Syrup
- 2 teaspoons Olive Oil
- 1/2 teaspoon Ground Cinnamon
- 1/2 teaspoon Pure Vanilla Extract
- 1/4 teaspoon Baking Powder
- 1/8 teaspoon Fine Sea Salt
- 1/4 cup Pecan Pieces, (1 ounce)

Directions:
1. Adjust the cooking rack to the bottom position and preheat toaster oven to 350°F on the BAKE setting. Grease a 7 x 5-inch toaster oven-safe baking dish.
2. In a large bowl, add the banana and mash well. Stir in the flaxseed meal, maple syrup, olive oil, cinnamon, vanilla, baking powder, salt, milk, oats, and pecan pieces. Pour mixture into prepared baking dish.
3. Bake oatmeal until the middle is set and browned on the edges, about 25 to 35 minutes. (For softer scoop able oatmeal bake 25 to 30 minutes, for firm oatmeal bake 30 to 35 minutes.)
4. Let sit at least 10 minutes before slicing and serving.

75. Chives Salmon And Shrimp Bowls

Servings: 4
Cooking Time: 12 Minutes
Ingredients:
- 1 pound shrimp, peeled and deveined
- ½ pound salmon fillets, boneless and cubed
- 2 spring onions, chopped
- 2 teaspoons olive oil
- 1 cup baby kale
- Salt and black pepper to the taste
- 1 tablespoon chives, chopped

Directions:
1. Preheat the air fryer with the oil at 330 degrees F, add the shrimp, salmon and the other ingredients, toss gently and cook for 12 minutes.
2. Divide everything into bowls and serve.
- **Nutrition Info:** calories 244, fat 11, fiber 4, carbs 5, protein 7

76. Simply Bacon

Servings: 1 Person
Cooking Time: 10 Minutes
Ingredients:
- 4 pieces of bacon

Directions:
1. Place the bacon strips on the instant vortex air fryer.
2. Cook for 10 minutes
3. at 200 degrees Celsius.
4. Check when it browns and shows to be ready. Serve.
- **Nutrition Info:** Calories 165, Fat 13g, Proteins 12 g, Carbs 0g

77. Herby Mushrooms With Vermouth

Servings: 4
Cooking Time: 20 Minutes
Ingredients:
- 2 lb portobello mushrooms, sliced
- 2 tbsp vermouth
- ½ tsp garlic powder
- 1 tbsp olive oil
- 2 tsp herbs
- 1 tbsp duck fat, softened

Directions:
1. Mix duck fat, garlic powder, and herbs in a bowl. Pour the mixture over the mushrooms and top with vermouth. Place the mushrooms in a baking dish and press Start. Cook for 15 minutes on Bake function at 350 F. Serve warm.

78. Crispy Tilapia Tacos

Servings: 4
Cooking Time: 5 Minutes
Ingredients:

- 2 tablespoons milk
- ⅓ cup mayonnaise
- ¼ teaspoon garlic powder
- 1 teaspoon chili powder
- 1½ cups panko bread crumbs
- ½ teaspoon salt
- 4 teaspoons canola oil
- 1 pound (454 g) skinless tilapia fillets, cut into 3-inch-long and 1-inch-wide strips
- 4 small flour tortillas
- Lemon wedges, for topping
- Cooking spray

Directions:
1. Spritz the air fryer basket with cooking spray.
2. Combine the milk, mayo, garlic powder, and chili powder in a bowl. Stir to mix well. Combine the panko with salt and canola oil in a separate bowl. Stir to mix well.
3. Dredge the tilapia strips in the milk mixture first, then dunk the strips in the panko mixture to coat well. Shake the excess off.
4. Arrange the tilapia strips in the pan.
5. Put the air fryer basket on the baking pan and slide into Rack Position 2, select Air Fry, set temperature to 400ºF (205ºC) and set time to 5 minutes.
6. Flip the strips halfway through the cooking time.
7. When cooking is complete, the strips will be opaque on all sides and the panko will be golden brown.
8. Unfold the tortillas on a large plate, then divide the tilapia strips over the tortillas. Squeeze the lemon wedges on top before serving.

LUNCH RECIPES

79. Zucchini Stew

Servings: 4
Cooking Time: 12 Minutes
Ingredients:
- 8 zucchinis, roughly cubed
- ¼ cup tomato sauce
- 1 tbsp. olive oil
- ½ tsp. basil; chopped.
- ¼ tsp. rosemary; dried
- Salt and black pepper to taste.

Directions:
1. Grease a pan that fits your air fryer with the oil, add all the ingredients, toss, introduce the pan in the fryer and cook at 350°F for 12 minutes
2. Divide into bowls and serve.
- **Nutrition Info:** Calories: 200; Fat: 6g; Fiber: 2g; Carbs: 4g; Protein: 6g

80. Beef Steaks With Beans

Servings: 4
Cooking Time: 10 Minutes
Ingredients:
- 4 beef steaks, trim the fat and cut into strips
- 1 cup green onions, chopped
- 2 cloves garlic, minced
- 1 red bell pepper, seeded and thinly sliced
- 1 can tomatoes, crushed
- 1 can cannellini beans
- 3/4 cup beef broth
- 1/4 teaspoon dried basil
- 1/2 teaspoon cayenne pepper
- 1/2 teaspoon sea salt
- 1/4 teaspoon ground black pepper, or to taste

Directions:
1. Preparing the ingredients. Add the steaks, green onions and garlic to the instant crisp air fryer basket.
2. Air frying. Close air fryer lid. Cook at 390 degrees f for 10 minutes, working in batches.
3. Stir in the remaining ingredients and cook for an additional 5 minutes.
- **Nutrition Info:** Calories 284 Total fat 7.9 g Saturated fat 1.4 g Cholesterol 36 mg Sodium 704 mg Total carbs 46 g Fiber 3.6 g Sugar 5.5 g Protein 17.9 g

81. Easy Italian Meatballs

Servings: 4
Cooking Time: 13 Minutes
Ingredients:
- 2-lb. lean ground turkey
- ¼ cup onion, minced
- 2 cloves garlic, minced
- 2 tablespoons parsley, chopped
- 2 eggs
- 1½ cup parmesan cheese, grated
- ½ teaspoon red pepper flakes
- ½ teaspoon Italian seasoning Salt and black pepper to taste

Directions:
1. Toss all the meatball Ingredients: in a bowl and mix well.
2. Make small meatballs out this mixture and place them in the air fryer basket.
3. Press "Power Button" of Air Fry Oven and turn the dial to select the "Air Fry" mode.
4. Press the Time button and again turn the dial to set the cooking time to 13 minutes.
5. Now push the Temp button and rotate the dial to set the temperature at 350 degrees F.
6. Once preheated, place the air fryer basket inside and close its lid.
7. Flip the meatballs when cooked halfway through.
8. Serve warm.
- **Nutrition Info:** Calories 472 Total Fat 25.8 g Saturated Fat .4 g Cholesterol 268 mg Sodium 503 mg Total Carbs 1.7 g Fiber 0.3 g Sugar 0.6 g Protein 59.6 g

82. Perfect Size French Fries

Servings: 1
Cooking Time: 30 Minutes
Ingredients:
- 1 medium potato
- 1 tablespoon olive oil
- Salt and pepper to taste

Directions:

1. Start by preheating your oven to 425°F.
2. Clean the potato and cut it into fries or wedges.
3. Place fries in a bowl of cold water to rinse.
4. Lay the fries on a thick sheet of paper towels and pat dry.
5. Toss in a bowl with oil, salt, and pepper.
6. Bake for 30 minutes.
- **Nutrition Info:** Calories: 284, Sodium: 13 mg, Dietary Fiber: 4.7 g, Total Fat: 14.2 g, Total Carbs: 37.3 g, Protein: 4.3 g.

83. Sweet Potato And Parsnip Spiralized Latkes

Servings: 12
Cooking Time: 20 Minutes
Ingredients:
- 1 medium sweet potato
- 1 large parsnip
- 4 cups water
- 1 egg + 1 egg white
- 2 scallions
- 1/2 teaspoon garlic powder
- 1/2 teaspoon sea salt
- 1/2 teaspoon ground pepper

Directions:
1. Start by spiralizing the sweet potato and parsnip and chopping the scallions, reserving only the green parts.
2. Preheat toaster oven to 425°F.
3. Bring 4 cups of water to a boil. Place all of your noodles in a colander and pour the boiling water over the top, draining well.
4. Let the noodles cool, then grab handfuls and place them in a paper towel; squeeze to remove as much liquid as possible.
5. In a large bowl, beat egg and egg white together. Add noodles, scallions, garlic powder, salt, and pepper, mix well.
6. Prepare a baking sheet; scoop out 1/4 cup of mixture at a time and place on sheet.
7. Slightly press down each scoop with your hands, then bake for 20 minutes, flipping halfway through.
- **Nutrition Info:** Calories: 24, Sodium: 91 mg, Dietary Fiber: 1.0 g, Total Fat: 0.4 g, Total Carbs: 4.3 g, Protein: 0.9 g.

84. Crispy Breaded Pork Chop

Servings: 6
Cooking Time: 12 Minutes
Ingredients:
- olive oil spray
- 6 3/4-inch thick center-cut boneless pork chops, fat trimmed (5 oz each)
- kosher salt
- 1 large egg, beaten
- 1/2 cup panko crumbs, check labels for GF
- 1/3 cup crushed cornflakes crumbs
- 2 tbsp grated parmesan cheese
- 1 1/4 tsp sweet paprika
- 1/2 tsp garlic powder
- 1/2 tsp onion powder
- 1/4 tsp chili powder
- 1/8 tsp black pepper

Directions:
1. Preheat the Instant Pot Duo Crisp Air Fryer for 12 minutes at 400°F.
2. On both sides, season pork chops with half teaspoon kosher salt.
3. Then combine cornflake crumbs, panko, parmesan cheese, 3/4 tsp kosher salt, garlic powder, paprika, onion powder, chili powder, and black pepper in a large bowl.
4. Place the egg beat in another bowl. Dip the pork in the egg & then crumb mixture.
5. When the air fryer is ready, place 3 of the chops into the Instant Pot Duo Crisp Air Fryer Basket and spritz the top with oil.
6. Close the Air Fryer lid and cook for 12 minutes turning halfway, spritzing both sides with oil.
7. Set aside and repeat with the remaining.
- **Nutrition Info:** Calories 281, Total Fat 13g, Total Carbs 8g, Protein 33g

85. Pumpkin Pancakes

Servings: 4
Cooking Time: 12 Minutes
Ingredients:
- 1 square puff pastry
- 3 tablespoons pumpkin filling
- 1 small egg, beaten

Directions:

1. Roll out a square of puff pastry and layer it with pumpkin pie filling, leaving about ¼-inch space around the edges.
2. Cut it up into 8 equal sized square pieces and coat the edges with beaten egg.
3. Press "Power Button" of Air Fry Oven and turn the dial to select the "Air Fry" mode.
4. Press the Time button and again turn the dial to set the cooking time to 12 minutes.
5. Now push the Temp button and rotate the dial to set the temperature at 355 degrees F.
6. Press "Start/Pause" button to start.
7. When the unit beeps to show that it is preheated, open the lid.
8. Arrange the squares into a greased "Sheet Pan" and insert in the oven.
9. Serve warm.
- **Nutrition Info:** Calories: 109 Cal Total Fat: 6.7 g Saturated Fat: 1.8 g Cholesterol: 34 mg Sodium: 87 mg Total Carbs: 9.8 g Fiber: 0.5 g Sugar: 2.6 g Protein: 2.4 g

86. Lobster Tails

Servings: 2
Cooking Time: 8 Minutes
Ingredients:
- 2 6oz lobster tails
- 1 tsp salt
- 1 tsp chopped chives
- 2 Tbsp unsalted butter melted
- 1 Tbsp minced garlic
- 1 tsp lemon juice

Directions:
1. Combine butter, garlic, salt, chives, and lemon juice to prepare butter mixture.
2. Butterfly lobster tails by cutting through shell followed by removing the meat and resting it on top of the shell.
3. Place them on the tray in the Instant Pot Duo Crisp Air Fryer basket and spread butter over the top of lobster meat. Close the Air Fryer lid, select the Air Fry option and cook on 380°F for 4 minutes.
4. Open the Air Fryer lid and spread more butter on top, cook for extra 2-4 minutes until done.
- **Nutrition Info:** Calories 120, Total Fat 12g, Total Carbs 2g, Protein 1g

87. Roasted Mini Peppers

Servings: 6
Cooking Time: 15 Minutes
Ingredients:
- 1 bag mini bell peppers
- Cooking spray
- Salt and pepper to taste

Directions:
1. Start by preheating toaster oven to 400°F.
2. Wash and dry the peppers, then place flat on a baking sheet.
3. Spray peppers with cooking spray and sprinkle with salt and pepper.
4. Roast for 15 minutes.
- **Nutrition Info:** Calories: 19, Sodium: 2 mg, Dietary Fiber: 1.3 g, Total Fat: 0.3 g, Total Carbs: 3.6 g, Protein: 0.6 g.

88. Air Fried Steak Sandwich

Servings: 4
Cooking Time: 16 Minutes
Ingredients:
- Large hoagie bun, sliced in half
- 6 ounces of sirloin or flank steak, sliced into bite-sized pieces
- ½ tablespoon of mustard powder
- ½ tablespoon of soy sauce
- 1 tablespoon of fresh bleu cheese, crumbled
- 8 medium-sized cherry tomatoes, sliced in half
- 1 cup of fresh arugula, rinsed and patted dry

Directions:
1. Preparing the ingredients. In a small mixing bowl, combine the soy sauce and onion powder; stir with a fork until thoroughly combined.
2. Lay the raw steak strips in the soy-mustard mixture, and fully immerse each piece to marinate.
3. Set the instant crisp air fryer to 320 degrees for 10 minutes.
4. Arrange the soy-mustard marinated steak pieces on a piece of tin foil, flat and not overlapping, and set the tin foil on one side of the instant crisp air fryer basket. The foil should not take up more than half of the surface.

5. Lay the hoagie-bun halves, crusty-side up and soft-side down, on the other half of the air-fryer.
6. Air frying. Close air fryer lid.
7. After 10 minutes, the instant crisp air fryer will shut off; the hoagie buns should be starting to crisp and the steak will have begun to cook.
8. Carefully, flip the hoagie buns so they are now crusty-side down and soft-side up; crumble a layer of the bleu cheese on each hoagie half.
9. With a long spoon, gently stir the marinated steak in the foil to ensure even coverage.
10. Set the instant crisp air fryer to 360 degrees for 6 minutes.
11. After 6 minutes, when the fryer shuts off, the bleu cheese will be perfectly melted over the toasted bread, and the steak will be juicy on the inside and crispy on the outside.
12. Remove the cheesy hoagie halves first, using tongs, and set on a serving plate; then cover one side with the steak, and top with the cherry-tomato halves and the arugula. Close with the other cheesy hoagie-half, slice into two pieces, and enjoy.
- **Nutrition Info:** Calories 284 Total fat 7.9 g Saturated fat 1.4 g Cholesterol 36 mg Sodium 704 mg Total carbs 46 g Fiber 3.6 g Sugar 5.5 g Protein 17.9 g

89. Skinny Black Bean Flautas

Servings: 10
Cooking Time: 25 Minutes
Ingredients:
- 2 (15-ounce) cans black beans
- 1 cup shredded cheddar
- 1 (4-ounce) can diced green chilies
- 2 teaspoons taco seasoning
- 10 (8-inch) whole wheat flour tortillas
- Olive oil

Directions:
1. Start by preheating toaster oven to 350°F.
2. Drain black beans and mash in a medium bowl with a fork.
3. Mix in cheese, chilies, and taco seasoning until all ingredients are thoroughly combined.
4. Evenly spread the mixture over each tortilla and wrap tightly.
5. Brush each side lightly with olive oil and place on a baking sheet.
6. Bake for 12 minutes, turn, and bake for another 13 minutes.
- **Nutrition Info:** Calories: 367, Sodium: 136 mg, Dietary Fiber: 14.4 g, Total Fat: 2.8 g, Total Carbs: 64.8 g, Protein: 22.6 g.

90. Turkey And Mushroom Stew

Servings: 4
Cooking Time: 12 Minutes
Ingredients:
- ½ lb. brown mushrooms; sliced
- 1 turkey breast, skinless, boneless; cubed and browned
- ¼ cup tomato sauce
- 1 tbsp. parsley; chopped.
- Salt and black pepper to taste.

Directions:
1. In a pan that fits your air fryer, mix the turkey with the mushrooms, salt, pepper and tomato sauce, toss, introduce in the fryer and cook at 350°F for 25 minutes
2. Divide into bowls and serve for lunch with parsley sprinkled on top.
- **Nutrition Info:** Calories: 220; Fat: 12g; Fiber: 2g; Carbs: 5g; Protein: 12g

91. Moroccan Pork Kebabs

Servings: 4
Cooking Time: 45 Minutes
Ingredients:
- 1/4 cup orange juice
- 1 tablespoon tomato paste
- 1 clove chopped garlic
- 1 tablespoon ground cumin
- 1/8 teaspoon ground cinnamon
- 4 tablespoons olive oil
- 1-1/2 teaspoons salt
- 3/4 teaspoon black pepper
- 1-1/2 pounds boneless pork loin
- 1 small eggplant
- 1 small red onion
- Pita bread (optional)
- 1/2 small cucumber
- 2 tablespoons chopped fresh mint

- Wooden skewers

Directions:
1. Start by placing wooden skewers in water to soak.
2. Cut pork loin and eggplant into 1- to 1-1/2-inch chunks.
3. Preheat toaster oven to 425°F.
4. Cut cucumber and onions into pieces and chop the mint.
5. In a large bowl, combine the orange juice, tomato paste, garlic, cumin, cinnamon, 2 tablespoons of oil, 1 teaspoon of salt, and 1/2 teaspoon of pepper.
6. Add the pork to this mixture and refrigerate for at least 30 minutes, but up to 8 hours.
7. Mix together vegetables, remaining oil, and salt and pepper.
8. Skewer the vegetables and bake for 20 minutes.
9. Add the pork to the skewers and bake for an additional 25 minutes.
10. Remove ingredients from skewers and sprinkle with mint; serve with flatbread if using.

- **Nutrition Info:** Calories: 465, Sodium: 1061 mg, Dietary Fiber: 5.6 g, Total Fat: 20.8 g, Total Carbs: 21.9 g, Protein: 48.2 g.

92. Spicy Avocado Cauliflower Toast

Servings: 2
Cooking Time: 15 Minutes
Ingredients:
- 1/2 large head of cauliflower, leaves removed
- 3 1/4 teaspoons olive oil
- 1 small jalapeño
- 1 tablespoon chopped cilantro leaves
- 2 slices whole grain bread
- 1 medium avocado
- Salt and pepper
- 5 radishes
- 1 green onion
- 2 teaspoons hot sauce
- 1 lime

Directions:
1. Start by preheating toaster oven to 450°F.
2. Cut cauliflower into thick pieces, about 3/4-inches-thick, and slice jalapeño into thin slices.
3. Place cauliflower and jalapeño in a bowl and mix together with 2 teaspoons olive oil.
4. Add salt and pepper to taste and mix for another minute.
5. Coat a pan with another teaspoon of olive oil, then lay the cauliflower mixture flat across the pan.
6. Cook for 20 minutes, flipping in the last 5 minutes.
7. Reduce heat to toast.
8. Sprinkle cilantro over the mix while it is still warm, and set aside.
9. Brush bread with remaining oil and toast until golden brown, about 5 minutes.
10. Dice onion and radish.
11. Mash avocado in a bowl, then spread on toast and sprinkle salt and pepper to taste.
12. Put cauliflower mix on toast and cover with onion and radish. Drizzle with hot sauce and serve with a lime wedge.

- **Nutrition Info:** Calories: 359, Sodium: 308 mg, Dietary Fiber: 11.1 g, Total Fat: 28.3 g, Total Carbs: 26.4 g, Protein: 6.6 g.

93. Spanish Chicken Bake

Servings: 4
Cooking Time: 25 Minutes
Ingredients:
- ½ onion, quartered
- ½ red onion, quartered
- ½ lb. potatoes, quartered
- 4 garlic cloves
- 4 tomatoes, quartered
- 1/8 cup chorizo
- ¼ teaspoon paprika powder
- 4 chicken thighs, boneless
- ¼ teaspoon dried oregano
- ½ green bell pepper, julienned
- Salt
- Black pepper

Directions:
1. Toss chicken, veggies, and all the Ingredients: in a baking tray.
2. Press "Power Button" of Air Fry Oven and turn the dial to select the "Bake" mode.

3. Press the Time button and again turn the dial to set the cooking time to 25 minutes.
4. Now push the Temp button and rotate the dial to set the temperature at 425 degrees F.
5. Once preheated, place the baking pan inside and close its lid.
6. Serve warm.
- **Nutrition Info:** Calories 301 Total Fat 8.9 g Saturated Fat 4.5 g Cholesterol 57 mg Sodium 340 mg Total Carbs 24.7 g Fiber 1.2 g Sugar 1.3 g Protein 15.3 g

94. Barbecue Air Fried Chicken

Servings: 10
Cooking Time: 26 Minutes
Ingredients:
- 1 teaspoon Liquid Smoke
- 2 cloves Fresh Garlic smashed
- 1/2 cup Apple Cider Vinegar
- 3 pounds Chuck Roast well-marbled with intramuscular fat
- 1 Tablespoon Kosher Salt
- 1 Tablespoon Freshly Ground Black Pepper
- 2 teaspoons Garlic Powder
- 1.5 cups Barbecue Sauce
- 1/4 cup Light Brown Sugar + more for sprinkling
- 2 Tablespoons Honey optional and in place of 2 TBL sugar

Directions:
1. Add meat to the Instant Pot Duo Crisp Air Fryer Basket, spreading out the meat.
2. Select the option Air Fry.
3. Close the Air Fryer lid and cook at 300 degrees F for 8 minutes. Pause the Air Fryer and flip meat over after 4 minutes.
4. Remove the lid and baste with more barbecue sauce and sprinkle with a little brown sugar.
5. Again Close the Air Fryer lid and set the temperature at 400°F for 9 minutes. Watch meat though the lid and flip it over after 5 minutes.
- **Nutrition Info:** Calories 360, Total Fat 16g, Total Carbs 27g, Protein 27g

95. Bok Choy And Butter Sauce(1)

Servings: 4
Cooking Time: 12 Minutes
Ingredients:
- 2 bok choy heads; trimmed and cut into strips
- 1 tbsp. butter; melted
- 2 tbsp. chicken stock
- 1 tsp. lemon juice
- 1 tbsp. olive oil
- A pinch of salt and black pepper

Directions:
1. In a pan that fits your air fryer, mix all the ingredients, toss, introduce the pan in the air fryer and cook at 380°F for 15 minutes.
2. Divide between plates and serve as a side dish
- **Nutrition Info:** Calories: 141; Fat: 3g; Fiber: 2g; Carbs: 4g; Protein: 3g

96. Mushroom Meatloaf

Servings: 4
Cooking Time: 25 Minutes
Ingredients:
- 14-ounce lean ground beef
- 1 chorizo sausage, chopped finely
- 1 small onion, chopped
- 1 garlic clove, minced
- 2 tablespoons fresh cilantro, chopped
- 3 tablespoons breadcrumbs
- 1 egg
- Salt and freshly ground black pepper, to taste
- 2 tablespoons fresh mushrooms, sliced thinly
- 3 tablespoons olive oil

Directions:
1. Preparing the ingredients. Preheat the instant crisp air fryer to 390 degrees f.
2. In a large bowl, add all ingredients except mushrooms and mix till well combined.
3. In a baking pan, place the beef mixture.
4. With the back of spatula, smooth the surface.
5. Top with mushroom slices and gently, press into the meatloaf.
6. Drizzle with oil evenly.
7. Air frying. Arrange the pan in the instant crisp air fryer basket, close air fryer lid and cook for about 25 minutes.

8. Cut the meatloaf in desires size wedges and serve.
- **Nutrition Info:** Calories 284 Total fat 7.9 g Saturated fat 1.4 g Cholesterol 36 mg Sodium 704 mg Total carbs 46 g Fiber 3.6 g Sugar 5.5 g Protein 17.9 g

97. Eggplant And Leeks Stew

Servings: 4
Cooking Time: 12 Minutes
Ingredients:
- 2 big eggplants, roughly cubed
- ½ bunch cilantro; chopped.
- 1 cup veggie stock
- 2 garlic cloves; minced
- 3 leeks; sliced
- 2 tbsp. olive oil
- 1 tbsp. hot sauce
- 1 tbsp. sweet paprika
- 1 tbsp. tomato puree
- Salt and black pepper to taste.

Directions:
1. In a pan that fits the air fryer, mix all the ingredients, toss, introduce in the fryer and cook at 380°F for 20 minutes
2. Divide the stew into bowls and serve for lunch.
- **Nutrition Info:** Calories: 183; Fat: 4g; Fiber: 2g; Carbs: 4g; Protein: 12g

98. Garlic Chicken Potatoes

Servings: 4
Cooking Time: 30 Minutes
Ingredients:
- 2 lbs. red potatoes, quartered
- 3 tablespoons olive oil
- 1/2 teaspoon cumin seeds
- Salt and black pepper, to taste
- 4 garlic cloves, chopped
- 2 tablespoons brown sugar
- 1 lemon (1/2 juiced and 1/2 cut into wedges)
- Pinch of red pepper flakes
- 4 skinless, boneless chicken breasts
- 2 tablespoons cilantro, chopped

Directions:
1. Place the chicken, lemon, garlic, and potatoes in a baking pan.
2. Toss the spices, herbs, oil, and sugar in a bowl.
3. Add this mixture to the chicken and veggies then toss well to coat.
4. Press "Power Button" of Air Fry Oven and turn the dial to select the "Bake" mode.
5. Press the Time button and again turn the dial to set the cooking time to 30 minutes.
6. Now push the Temp button and rotate the dial to set the temperature at 400 degrees F.
7. Once preheated, place the baking pan inside and close its lid.
8. Serve warm.
- **Nutrition Info:** Calories 545 Total Fat 36.4 g Saturated Fat 10.1 g Cholesterol 200 mg Sodium 272 mg Total Carbs 40.7 g Fiber 0.2 g Sugar 0.1 g Protein 42.5 g

99. Turkey-stuffed Peppers

Servings: 6
Cooking Time: 35 Minutes
Ingredients:
- 1 pound lean ground turkey
- 1 tablespoon olive oil
- 2 cloves garlic, minced
- 1/3 onion, minced
- 1 tablespoon cilantro (optional)
- 1 teaspoon garlic powder
- 1 teaspoon cumin powder
- 1/2 teaspoon salt
- Pepper to taste
- 3 large red bell peppers
- 1 cup chicken broth
- 1/4 cup tomato sauce
- 1-1/2 cups cooked brown rice
- 1/4 cup shredded cheddar
- 6 green onions

Directions:
1. Start by preheating toaster oven to 400°F.
2. Heat a skillet on medium heat.
3. Add olive oil to the skillet, then mix in onion and garlic.
4. Sauté for about 5 minutes, or until the onion starts to look opaque.
5. Add the turkey to the skillet and season with cumin, garlic powder, salt, and pepper.
6. Brown the meat until thoroughly cooked, then mix in chicken broth and tomato sauce.

7. Reduce heat and simmer for about 5 minutes, stirring occasionally.
8. Add the brown rice and continue stirring until it is evenly spread through the mix.
9. Cut the bell peppers lengthwise down the middle and remove all of the seeds.
10. Grease a pan or line it with parchment paper and lay all peppers in the pan with the outside facing down.
11. Spoon the meat mixture evenly into each pepper and use the back of the spoon to level.
12. Bake for 30 minutes.
13. Remove pan from oven and sprinkle cheddar over each pepper, then put it back in for another 3 minutes, or until the cheese is melted.
14. While the cheese melts, dice the green onions. Remove pan from oven and sprinkle onions over each pepper and serve.
- **Nutrition Info:** Calories: 394, Sodium: 493 mg, Dietary Fiber: 4.1 g, Total Fat: 12.9 g, Total Carbs: 44.4 g, Protein: 27.7 g.

100. Fried Whole Chicken

Servings: 4
Cooking Time: 70 Minutes
Ingredients:
- 1 Whole chicken
- 2 Tbsp or spray of oil of choice
- 1 tsp garlic powder
- 1 tsp onion powder
- 1 tsp paprika
- 1 tsp Italian seasoning
- 2 Tbsp Montreal Steak Seasoning (or salt and pepper to taste)
- 1.5 cup chicken broth

Directions:
1. Truss and wash the chicken.
2. Mix the seasoning and rub a little amount on the chicken.
3. Pour the broth inside the Instant Pot Duo Crisp Air Fryer.
4. Place the chicken in the air fryer basket.
5. Select the option Air Fry and Close the Air Fryer lid and cook for 25 minutes.
6. Spray or rub the top of the chicken with oil and rub it with half of the seasoning.
7. Close the air fryer lid and air fry again at 400°F for 10 minutes.
8. Flip the chicken, spray it with oil, and rub with the remaining seasoning.
9. Again air fry it for another ten minutes.
10. Allow the chicken to rest for 10 minutes.
- **Nutrition Info:** Calories 436, Total Fat 28g, Total Carbs 4g, Protein 42g

101. Seven-layer Tostadas

Servings: 6
Cooking Time: 5 Minutes
Ingredients:
- 1 (16-ounce) can refried pinto beans
- 1-1/2 cups guacamole
- 1 cup light sour cream
- 1/2 teaspoon taco seasoning
- 1 cup shredded Mexican cheese blend
- 1 cup chopped tomatoes
- 1/2 cup thinly sliced green onions
- 1/2 cup sliced black olives
- 6-8 whole wheat flour tortillas small enough to fit in your oven
- Olive oil

Directions:
1. Start by placing baking sheet into toaster oven while preheating it to 450°F. Remove pan and drizzle with olive oil.
2. Place tortillas on pan and cook in oven until they are crisp, turn at least once, this should take about 5 minutes or less.
3. In a medium bowl, mash refried beans to break apart any chunks, then microwave for 2 1/2 minutes.
4. Stir taco seasoning into the sour cream. Chop vegetables and halve olives.
5. Top tortillas with ingredients in this order: refried beans, guacamole, sour cream, shredded cheese, tomatoes, onions, and olives.
- **Nutrition Info:** Calories: 657, Sodium: 581 mg, Dietary Fiber: 16.8 g, Total Fat: 31.7 g, Total Carbs: 71.3 g, Protein: 28.9 g.

102. Parmesan Chicken Meatballs

Servings: 4
Cooking Time: 12 Minutes
Ingredients:

- 1-lb. ground chicken
- 1 large egg, beaten
- ½ cup Parmesan cheese, grated
- ½ cup pork rinds, ground
- 1 teaspoon garlic powder
- 1 teaspoon paprika
- 1 teaspoon kosher salt
- ½ teaspoon pepper
- Crust:
- ½ cup pork rinds, ground

Directions:
1. Toss all the meatball Ingredients: in a bowl and mix well.
2. Make small meatballs out this mixture and roll them in the pork rinds.
3. Place the coated meatballs in the air fryer basket.
4. Press "Power Button" of Air Fry Oven and turn the dial to select the "Bake" mode.
5. Press the Time button and again turn the dial to set the cooking time to 12 minutes.
6. Now push the Temp button and rotate the dial to set the temperature at 400 degrees F.
7. Once preheated, place the air fryer basket inside and close its lid.
8. Serve warm.
- **Nutrition Info:** Calories 529 Total Fat 17 g Saturated Fat 3 g Cholesterol 65 mg Sodium 391 mg Total Carbs 55 g Fiber 6 g Sugar 8 g Protein 41g

103. Sweet & Sour Pork

Servings: 4
Cooking Time: 27 Minutes
Ingredients:
- 2 pounds Pork cut into chunks
- 2 large Eggs
- 1 teaspoon Pure Sesame Oil (optional)
- 1 cup Potato Starch (or cornstarch)
- 1/2 teaspoon Sea Salt
- 1/4 teaspoon Freshly Ground Black Pepper
- 1/16 teaspoon Chinese Five Spice
- 3 Tablespoons Canola Oil
- Oil Mister

Directions:
1. In a mixing bowl, combine salt, potato starch, Chinese Five Spice, and peppers.
2. In another bowl, beat the eggs & add sesame oil.
3. Then dredge the pieces of Pork into the Potato Starch and remove the excess. Then dip each piece into the egg mixture, shake off excess, and then back into the Potato Starch mixture.
4. Place pork pieces into the Instant Pot Duo Crisp Air Fryer Basket after spray the pork with oil.
5. Close the Air Fryer lid and cook at 340°F for approximately 8 to 12 minutes (or until pork is cooked), shaking the basket a couple of times for evenly distribution.
- **Nutrition Info:** Calories 521, Total Fat 21g, Total Carbs 23g, Protein 60g

104. Pork Stew

Servings: 4
Cooking Time: 12 Minutes
Ingredients:
- 2 lb. pork stew meat; cubed
- 1 eggplant; cubed
- ½ cup beef stock
- 2 zucchinis; cubed
- ½ tsp. smoked paprika
- Salt and black pepper to taste.
- A handful cilantro; chopped.

Directions:
1. In a pan that fits your air fryer, mix all the ingredients, toss, introduce in your air fryer and cook at 370°F for 30 minutes
2. Divide into bowls and serve right away.
- **Nutrition Info:** Calories: 245; Fat: 12g; Fiber: 2g; Carbs: 5g; Protein: 14g

105. Turkey Meatballs With Manchego Cheese

Servings: 4
Cooking Time: 10 Minutes
Ingredients:
- 1 pound ground turkey
- 1/2 pound ground pork
- 1 egg, well beaten
- 1 teaspoon dried basil
- 1 teaspoon dried rosemary
- 1/4 cup Manchego cheese, grated
- 2 tablespoons yellow onions, finely chopped

- 1 teaspoon fresh garlic, finely chopped
- Sea salt and ground black pepper, to taste

Directions:
1. In a mixing bowl, combine all the ingredients until everything is well incorporated.
2. Shape the mixture into 1-inch balls.
3. Cook the meatballs in the preheated Air Fryer at 380 degrees for 7 minutes. Shake halfway through the cooking time. Work in batches.
4. Serve with your favorite pasta.
- **Nutrition Info:** 386 Calories; 24g Fat; 9g Carbs; 41g Protein; 3g Sugars; 2g Fiber

106. Okra Casserole

Servings: 4
Cooking Time: 12 Minutes
Ingredients:
- 2 red bell peppers; cubed
- 2 tomatoes; chopped.
- 3 garlic cloves; minced
- 3 cups okra
- ½ cup cheddar; shredded
- ¼ cup tomato puree
- 1 tbsp. cilantro; chopped.
- 1 tsp. olive oil
- 2 tsp. coriander, ground
- Salt and black pepper to taste.

Directions:
1. Grease a heat proof dish that fits your air fryer with the oil, add all the ingredients except the cilantro and the cheese and toss them really gently
2. Sprinkle the cheese and the cilantro on top, introduce the dish in the fryer and cook at 390°F for 20 minutes.
3. Divide between plates and serve for lunch.
- **Nutrition Info:** Calories: 221; Fat: 7g; Fiber: 2g; Carbs: 4g; Protein: 9g

107. Persimmon Toast With Sour Cream & Cinnamon

Servings: 1
Cooking Time: 5 Minutes
Ingredients:
- 1 slice of wheat bread
- 1/2 persimmon
- Sour cream to taste
- Sugar to taste
- Cinnamon to taste

Directions:
1. Spread a thin layer of sour cream across the bread.
2. Slice the persimmon into 1/4 inch pieces and lay them across the bread.
3. Sprinkle cinnamon and sugar over persimmon.
4. Toast in toaster oven until bread and persimmon begin to brown.
- **Nutrition Info:** Calories: 89, Sodium: 133 mg, Dietary Fiber: 2.0 g, Total Fat: 1.1 g, Total Carbs: 16.5 g, Protein: 3.8 g.

108. Okra And Green Beans Stew

Servings: 4
Cooking Time: 12 Minutes
Ingredients:
- 1 lb. green beans; halved
- 4 garlic cloves; minced
- 1 cup okra
- 3 tbsp. tomato sauce
- 1 tbsp. thyme; chopped.
- Salt and black pepper to taste.

Directions:
1. In a pan that fits your air fryer, mix all the ingredients, toss, introduce the pan in the air fryer and cook at 370°F for 15 minutes
2. Divide the stew into bowls and serve.
- **Nutrition Info:** Calories: 183; Fat: 5g; Fiber: 2g; Carbs: 4g; Protein: 8g

109. Air Fried Sausages

Servings: 6
Cooking Time: 13 Minutes
Ingredients:
- 6 sausage
- olive oil spray

Directions:
1. Pour 5 cup of water into Instant Pot Duo Crisp Air Fryer. Place air fryer basket inside the pot, spray inside with nonstick spray and put sausage links inside.
2. Close the Air Fryer lid and steam for about 5 minutes.

3. Remove the lid once done. Spray links with olive oil and close air crisp lid.
4. Set to air crisp at 400°F for 8 min flipping halfway through so both sides get browned.
- **Nutrition Info:** Calories 267, Total Fat 23g, Total Carbs 2g, Protein 13g

110. Vegetarian Philly Sandwich

Servings: 2
Cooking Time: 20 Minutes
Ingredients:
- 2 tablespoons olive oil
- 8 ounces sliced portabello mushrooms
- 1 vidalia onion, thinly sliced
- 1 green bell pepper, thinly sliced
- 1 red bell pepper, thinly sliced
- Salt and pepper
- 4 slices 2% provolone cheese
- 4 rolls

Directions:
1. Preheat toaster oven to 475°F.
2. Heat the oil in a medium sauce pan over medium heat.
3. Sauté mushrooms about 5 minutes, then add the onions and peppers and sauté another 10 minutes.
4. Slice rolls lengthwise and divide the vegetables into each roll.
5. Add the cheese and toast until the rolls start to brown and the cheese melts.
- **Nutrition Info:** Calories: 645, Sodium: 916 mg, Dietary Fiber: 7.2 g, Total Fat: 33.3 g, Total Carbs: 61.8 g, Protein: 27.1 g.

111. Coconut Shrimp With Dip

Servings: 4
Cooking Time: 9 Minutes
Ingredients:
- 1 lb large raw shrimp peeled and deveined with tail on
- 2 eggs beaten
- ¼ cup Panko Breadcrumbs
- 1 tsp salt
- ¼ tsp black pepper
- ½ cup All-Purpose Flour
- ½ cup unsweetened shredded coconut
- Oil for spraying

Directions:
1. Clean and dry the shrimp. Set it aside.
2. Take 3 bowls. Put flour in the first bowl. Beat eggs in the second bowl. Mix coconut, breadcrumbs, salt, and black pepper in the third bowl.
3. Select the Air Fry option and adjust the temperature to 390°F. Push start and preheating will start.
4. Dip each shrimp in flour followed by the egg and then coconut mixture, ensuring shrimp is covered on all sides during each dip.
5. Once the preheating is done, place shrimp in a single layer on greased tray in the basket of the Instant Pot Duo Crisp Air Fryer.
6. Spray the shrimp with oil lightly, and then close the Air Fryer basket lid. Cook for around 4 minutes.
7. After 4 minutes
8. open the Air Fryer basket lid and flip the shrimp over. Respray the shrimp with oil, close the Air Fryer basket lid, and cook for five more minutes.
9. Remove shrimp from the basket and serve with Thai Sweet Chili Sauce.
- **Nutrition Info:** Calories 279, Total Fat 11g, Total Carbs 17g, Protein 28g

112. Kale And Pine Nuts

Servings: 4
Cooking Time: 12 Minutes
Ingredients:
- 10 cups kale; torn
- 1/3 cup pine nuts
- 2 tbsp. lemon zest; grated
- 1 tbsp. lemon juice
- 2 tbsp. olive oil
- Salt and black pepper to taste.

Directions:
1. In a pan that fits the air fryer, combine all the ingredients, toss, introduce the pan in the machine and cook at 380°F for 15 minutes
2. Divide between plates and serve as a side dish.
- **Nutrition Info:** Calories: 121; Fat: 9g; Fiber: 2g; Carbs: 4g; Protein: 5g

113. Chicken With Veggies And Rice

Servings: 3
Cooking Time: 20 Minutes
Ingredients:
- 3 cups cold boiled white rice
- 1 cup cooked chicken, diced
- ½ cup frozen carrots
- ½ cup frozen peas
- ½ cup onion, chopped
- 6 tablespoons soy sauce
- 1 tablespoon vegetable oil

Directions:
1. Preheat the Air fryer to 360 degree F and grease a 7" nonstick pan.
2. Mix the rice, soy sauce, and vegetable oil in a bowl.
3. Stir in the remaining ingredients and mix until well combined.
4. Transfer the rice mixture into the pan and place in the Air fryer.
5. Cook for about 20 minutes and dish out to serve immediately.
- **Nutrition Info:** Calories: 405, Fat: 6.4g, Carbohydrates: 63g, Sugar: 3.5g, Protein: 21.7g, Sodium: 1500mg

114. Rolled Salmon Sandwich

Servings: 1
Cooking Time: 5 Minutes
Ingredients:
- 1 piece of flatbread
- 1 salmon filet
- Pinch of salt
- 1 tablespoon green onion, chopped
- 1/4 teaspoon dried sumac
- 1/2 teaspoon thyme
- 1/2 teaspoon sesame seeds
- 1/4 English cucumber
- 1 tablespoon yogurt

Directions:
1. Start by peeling and chopping the cucumber. Cut the salmon at a 45-degree angle into 4 slices and lay them flat on the flatbread.
2. Sprinkle salmon with salt to taste. Sprinkle onions, thyme, sumac, and sesame seeds evenly over the salmon.
3. Broil the salmon for at least 3 minutes, but longer if you want a more well-done fish.
4. While you broil your salmon, mix together the yogurt and cucumber. Remove your flatbread from the toaster oven and put it on a plate, then spoon the yogurt mix over the salmon.
5. Fold the sides of the flatbread in and roll it up for a gourmet lunch that you can take on the go.
- **Nutrition Info:** Calories: 347, Sodium: 397 mg, Dietary Fiber: 1.6 g, Total Fat: 12.4 g, Total Carbs: 20.6 g, Protein: 38.9 g.

115. Turkey Meatloaf

Servings: 4
Cooking Time: 20 Minutes
Ingredients:
- 1 pound ground turkey
- 1 cup kale leaves, trimmed and finely chopped
- 1 cup onion, chopped
- ½ cup fresh breadcrumbs
- 1 cup Monterey Jack cheese, grated
- 2 garlic cloves, minced
- ¼ cup salsa verde
- 1 teaspoon red chili powder
- ½ teaspoon ground cumin
- ½ teaspoon dried oregano, crushed
- Salt and ground black pepper, as required

Directions:
1. Preheat the Air fryer to 400 degree F and grease an Air fryer basket.
2. Mix all the ingredients in a bowl and divide the turkey mixture into 4 equal-sized portions.
3. Shape each into a mini loaf and arrange the loaves into the Air fryer basket.
4. Cook for about 20 minutes and dish out to serve warm.
- **Nutrition Info:** Calories: 435, Fat: 23.1g, Carbohydrates: 18.1g, Sugar: 3.6g, Protein: 42.2g, Sodium: 641mg

116. Spicy Green Crusted Chicken

Servings: 6
Cooking Time: 40 Minutes
Ingredients:

- 6 eggs, beaten
- 6 teaspoons parsley
- 4 teaspoons thyme
- 1 pound chicken pieces
- 6 teaspoons oregano
- Salt and freshly ground black pepper, to taste
- 4 teaspoons paprika

Directions:
1. Preheat the Air fryer to 360 degree F and grease an Air fryer basket.
2. Whisk eggs in a bowl and mix all the ingredients in another bowl except chicken pieces.
3. Dip the chicken in eggs and then coat generously with the dry mixture.
4. Arrange half of the chicken pieces in the Air fryer basket and cook for about 20 minutes.
5. Repeat with the remaining mixture and dish out to serve hot.
- **Nutrition Info:** Calories: 218, Fat: 10.4g, Carbohydrates: 2.6g, Sugar: 0.6g, Protein: 27.9g, Sodium: 128mg

117. Lamb Gyro

Servings: 4
Cooking Time: 25 Minutes
Ingredients:
- 1 pound ground lamb
- ¼ red onion, minced
- ¼ cup mint, minced
- ¼ cup parsley, minced
- 2 cloves garlic, minced
- ½ teaspoon salt
- ⅛ teaspoon rosemary
- ½ teaspoon black pepper
- 4 slices pita bread
- ¾ cup hummus
- 1 cup romaine lettuce, shredded
- ½ onion sliced
- 1 Roma tomato, diced
- ½ cucumber, skinned and thinly sliced
- 12 mint leaves, minced
- Tzatziki sauce, to taste

Directions:
1. Mix ground lamb, red onion, mint, parsley, garlic, salt, rosemary, and black pepper until fully incorporated.
2. Select the Broil function on the COSORI Air Fryer Toaster Oven, set time to 25 minutes and temperature to 450°F, then press Start/Cancel to preheat.
3. Line the food tray with parchment paper and place ground lamb on top, shaping it into a patty 1-inch-thick and 6 inches in diameter.
4. Insert the food tray at top position in the preheated air fryer toaster oven, then press Start/Cancel.
5. Remove when done and cut into thin slices.
6. Assemble each gyro starting with pita bread, then hummus, lamb meat, lettuce, onion, tomato, cucumber, and mint leaves, then drizzle with tzatziki.
7. Serve immediately.
- **Nutrition Info:** Calories: 409 kcal Total Fat: 14.6 g Saturated Fat: 0 g Cholesterol: 0 mg Sodium: 0 mg Total Carbs: 29.9 g Fiber: 0 g Sugar: 0 g Protein: 39.4 g

DINNER RECIPES

118. Herbed Eggplant

Servings: 2
Cooking Time: 15 Minutes
Ingredients:
- 1 large eggplant, cubed
- ½ teaspoon dried marjoram, crushed
- ½ teaspoon dried oregano, crushed
- ½ teaspoon dried thyme, crushed
- ½ teaspoon garlic powder
- Salt and black pepper, to taste
- Olive oil cooking spray

Directions:
1. Preheat the Air fryer to 390 degree F and grease an Air fryer basket.
2. Mix herbs, garlic powder, salt, and black pepper in a bowl.
3. Spray the eggplant cubes with cooking spray and rub with the herb mixture.
4. Arrange the eggplant cubes in the Air fryer basket and cook for about 15 minutes, flipping twice in between.
5. Dish out onto serving plates and serve hot.
- **Nutrition Info:** Calories: 62, Fat: 0.5g, Carbohydrates: 14.5g, Sugar: 7.1g, Protein: 2.4g, Sodium: 83mg

119. Lemon Duck Legs

Servings: 6
Cooking Time: 25 Minutes
Ingredients:
- 1 lemon
- 2-pound duck legs
- 1 teaspoon ground coriander
- 1 teaspoon ground nutmeg
- 1 teaspoon kosher salt
- ½ teaspoon dried rosemary
- 1 tablespoon olive oil
- 1 teaspoon stevia extract
- ¼ teaspoon sage

Directions:
1. Squeeze the juice from the lemon and grate the zest.
2. Combine the lemon juice and lemon zest together in the big mixing bowl.
3. Add the ground coriander, ground nutmeg, kosher salt, dried rosemary, and sage.
4. Sprinkle the liquid with the olive oil and stevia extract.
5. Whisk it carefully and put the duck legs there.
6. Stir the duck legs and leave them for 15 minutes to marinate.
7. Meanwhile, preheat the air fryer to 380 F.
8. Put the marinated duck legs in the air fryer and cook them for 25 minutes.
9. Turn the duck legs into another side after 15 minutes of cooking.
10. When the duck legs are cooked – let them cool little.
11. Serve and enjoy!
- **Nutrition Info:** calories 296, fat 11.5, fiber 0.5, carbs 1.6, protein 44.2

120. Shrimp Kebabs

Servings: 2
Cooking Time: 10 Minutes
Ingredients:
- ¾ pound shrimp, peeled and deveined
- 1 tablespoon fresh cilantro, chopped
- Wooden skewers, presoaked
- 2 tablespoons fresh lemon juice
- 1 teaspoon garlic, minced
- ½ teaspoon paprika
- ½ teaspoon ground cumin
- Salt and ground black pepper, as required

Directions:
1. Preheat the Air fryer to 350 degree F and grease an Air fryer basket.
2. Mix lemon juice, garlic, and spices in a bowl.
3. Stir in the shrimp and mix to coat well.
4. Thread the shrimp onto presoaked wooden skewers and transfer to the Air fryer basket.
5. Cook for about 10 minutes, flipping once in between.
6. Dish out the mixture onto serving plates and serve garnished with fresh cilantro.
- **Nutrition Info:** Calories: 212, Fat: 3.2g, Carbohydrates: 3.9g, Sugar: 0.4g, Protein: 39.1g, Sodium: 497mg

121. Delicious Beef Roast With Red Potatoes

Servings: 3
Cooking Time: 25 Minutes
Ingredients:
- 2 tbsp olive oil
- 4 pound top round roast beef
- 1 tsp salt
- ¼ tsp fresh ground black pepper
- 1 tsp dried thyme
- ½ tsp fresh rosemary, chopped
- 3 pounds red potatoes, halved
- Olive oil, black pepper and salt for garnish

Directions:
1. Preheat your Air Fryer to 360 F. In a small bowl, mix rosemary, salt, pepper and thyme; rub oil onto beef. Season with the spice mixture. Place the prepared meat in your Air Fryer's cooking basket and cook for 20 minutes.
2. Give the meat a turn and add potatoes, more pepper and oil. Cook for 20 minutes more. Take the steak out and set aside to cool for 10 minutes. Cook the potatoes in your Air Fryer for 10 more minutes at 400 F. Serve hot.
- **Nutrition Info:** 346 Calories; 11g Fat; 4g Carbs; 32g Protein; 1g Sugars; 1g Fiber

122. Air Fryer Veggie Quesdillas

Servings: 4
Cooking Time: 40 Minutes
Ingredients:
- 4 sprouted whole-grain flour tortillas (6-in.)
- 1 cup sliced red bell pepper
- 4 ounces reduced-fat Cheddar cheese, shredded
- 1 cup sliced zucchini
- 1 cup canned black beans, drained and rinsed (no salt)
- Cooking spray
- 2 ounces plain 2% reduced-fat Greek yogurt
- 1 teaspoon lime zest
- 1 Tbsp. fresh juice (from 1 lime)
- ¼ tsp. ground cumin
- 2 tablespoons chopped fresh cilantro
- 1/2 cup drained refrigerated pico de gallo

Directions:
1. Place tortillas on work surface, sprinkle 2 tablespoons shredded cheese over half of each tortilla and top with cheese on each tortilla with 1/4 cup each red pepper slices, zucchini slices, and black beans. Sprinkle evenly with remaining 1/2 cup cheese.
2. Fold tortillas over to form half-moon shaped quesadillas, lightly coat with cooking spray, and secure with toothpicks.
3. Lightly spray air fryer basket with cooking spray. Place 2 quesadillas in the basket, and cook at 400°F for 10 minutes until tortillas are golden brown and slightly crispy, cheese is melted, and vegetables are slightly softened. Turn quesadillas over halfway through cooking.
4. Repeat with remaining quesadillas.
5. Meanwhile, stir yogurt, lime juice, lime zest and cumin in a small bowl.
6. Cut each quesadilla into wedges and sprinkle with cilantro.
7. Serve with 1 tablespoon cumin cream and 2 tablespoons pico de gallo each.
- **Nutrition Info:** Calories 291 Fat 8g Saturated fat 4g Unsaturated fat 3g Protein 17g Carbohydrate 36g Fiber 8g Sugars 3g Sodium 518mg Calcium 30% DV Potassium 6% DV

123. Coconut Crusted Shrimp

Servings: 3
Cooking Time: 40 Minutes
Ingredients:
- 8 ounces coconut milk
- ½ cup sweetened coconut, shredded
- ½ cup panko breadcrumbs
- 1 pound large shrimp, peeled and deveined
- Salt and black pepper, to taste

Directions:
1. Preheat the Air fryer to 350-degree F and grease an Air fryer basket.
2. Place the coconut milk in a shallow bowl.
3. Mix coconut, breadcrumbs, salt, and black pepper in another bowl.
4. Dip each shrimp into coconut milk and finally, dredge in the coconut mixture.

5. Arrange half of the shrimps into the Air fryer basket and cook for about 20 minutes.
6. Dish out the shrimps onto serving plates and repeat with the remaining mixture to serve.
- **Nutrition Info:** Calories: 408, Fats: 23.7g, Carbohydrates: 11.7g, Sugar: 3.4g, Proteins: 31g, Sodium: 253mg

124. Miso-glazed Salmon

Servings: 4
Cooking Time: 5 Minutes
Ingredients:
- 1/4 cup red or white miso
- 1/3 cup sake
- 1 tablespoon soy sauce
- 2 tablespoons vegetable oil
- 1/4 cup sugar
- 4 skinless salmon filets

Directions:
1. In a shallow bowl, mix together the miso, sake, oil, soy sauce, and sugar.
2. Toss the salmon in the mixture until thoroughly coated on all sides.
3. Preheat your toaster oven to "high" on broil mode.
4. Place salmon in a broiling pan and broil until the top is well charred—about 5 minutes.
- **Nutrition Info:** Calories: 401, Sodium: 315 mg, Dietary Fiber: 0 g, Total Fat: 19.2 g, Total Carbs: 14.1 g, Protein: 39.2 g.

125. Couscous Stuffed Tomatoes

Servings: 4
Cooking Time: 25 Minutes
Ingredients:
- 4 tomatoes, tops and seeds removed
- 1 parsnip, peeled and finely chopped
- 1 cup mushrooms, chopped
- 1½ cups couscous
- 1 teaspoon olive oil
- 1 garlic clove, minced
- 1 tablespoon mirin sauce

Directions:
1. Preheat the Air fryer to 355 degree F and grease an Air fryer basket.
2. Heat olive oil in a skillet on low heat and add parsnips, mushrooms and garlic.
3. Cook for about 5 minutes and stir in the mirin sauce and couscous.
4. Stuff the couscous mixture into the tomatoes and arrange into the Air fryer basket.
5. Cook for about 20 minutes and dish out to serve warm.
- **Nutrition Info:** Calories: 361, Fat: 2g, Carbohydrates: 75.5g, Sugar: 5.1g, Protein: 10.4g, Sodium: 37mg

126. Shrimps, Zucchini, And Tomatoes On The Grill

Servings: 2
Cooking Time: 15 Minutes
Ingredients:
- 10 jumbo shrimps, peeled and deveined
- Salt and pepper to taste
- 1 clove of garlic, minced
- 1 medium zucchini, sliced
- 1-pint cherry tomatoes
- ¼ cup feta cheese

Directions:
1. Place the instant pot air fryer lid on and preheat the instant pot at 390 degrees F.
2. Place the grill pan accessory in the instant pot.
3. In a mixing bowl, season the shrimps with salt and pepper. Stir in the garlic, zucchini, and tomatoes.
4. Place on the grill pan, close the air fryer lid and cook for 15 minutes.
5. Once cooked, transfer to a bowl and sprinkle with feta cheese.
- **Nutrition Info:** Calories: 257; Carbs:4.2 g; Protein: 48.9g; Fat: 5.3g

127. Spicy Cauliflower Rice

Servings: 2
Cooking Time: 22 Minutes
Ingredients:
- 1 cauliflower head, cut into florets 1/2 tsp cumin
- 1/2 tsp chili powder
- 6 onion spring, chopped 2 jalapenos, chopped

- 4 tbsp olive oil
- 1 zucchini, trimmed and cut into cubes 1/2 tsp paprika
- 1/2 tsp garlic powder 1/2 tsp cayenne pepper 1/2 tsp pepper
- 1/2 tsp salt

Directions:
1. Preheat the air fryer to 370 F.
2. Add cauliflower florets into the food processor and process until it looks like rice.
3. Transfer cauliflower rice into the air fryer baking pan and drizzle with half oil.
4. Place pan in the air fryer and cook for 12 minutes, stir halfway through.
5. Heat remaining oil in a small pan over medium heat.
6. Add zucchini and cook for 5-8 minutes.
7. Add onion and jalapenos and cook for 5 minutes.
8. Add spices and stir well. Set aside.
9. Add cauliflower rice in the zucchini mixture and stir well.
10. Serve and enjoy.
- **Nutrition Info:** Calories 254 Fat 28 g Carbohydrates 12.3 g Sugar 5 g

128. Rigatoni With Roasted Broccoli And Chick Peas

Servings: 4
Cooking Time: 10 Minutes
Ingredients:
- 1 can anchovies packed in oil
- 4 cloves garlic, chopped
- 1 can chickpeas
- 1 chicken bouillon cube
- 1 pound broccoli, cut into small florets
- 1/2 pound whole wheat rigatoni
- 1/2 cup grated Romano cheese

Directions:
1. Drain and chop anchovies (set aside oil for later use), and cut broccoli into small florets.
2. Preheat toaster oven to 450°F.
3. In a shallow sauce pan, sauté anchovies in their oil, with garlic, until the garlic browns.
4. Drain the chickpeas, saving the canned liquid.
5. Add the chickpea liquid and bouillon to the anchovies, stir until bouillon dissolves.
6. Pour anchovy mix into a roasting pan and add broccoli and chickpeas.
7. Roast for 20 minutes.
8. While the veggies roast, cook rigatoni per package directions; drain the pasta, saving one cup of water.
9. Add the pasta to the anchovy mix and roast for another 10 minutes. Add reserved water, stirring in a little at a time until the pasta reaches the desired consistency.
10. Top with Romano and serve.
- **Nutrition Info:** Calories: 574, Sodium: 1198 mg, Dietary Fiber: 13.7 g, Total Fat: 14.0 g, Total Carbs: 81.1 g, Protein: 31.1 g.

129. Chargrilled Halibut Niçoise With Vegetables

Servings: 6
Cooking Time: 15 Minutes
Ingredients:
- 1 ½ pounds halibut fillets
- Salt and pepper to taste
- 2 tablespoons olive oil
- 2 pounds mixed vegetables
- 4 cups torn lettuce leaves
- 1 cup cherry tomatoes, halved
- 4 large hard-boiled eggs, peeled and sliced

Directions:
1. Place the instant pot air fryer lid on and preheat the instant pot at 390 degrees F.
2. Place the grill pan accessory in the instant pot.
3. Rub the halibut with salt and pepper. Brush the fish with oil.
4. Place on the grill.
5. Surround the fish fillet with the mixed vegetables, close the air fryer lid and grill for 15 minutes.
6. Assemble the salad by serving the fish fillet with mixed grilled vegetables, lettuce, cherry tomatoes, and hard-boiled eggs.
- **Nutrition Info:** Calories: 312; Carbs:16.8 g; Protein: 19.8g; Fat: 18.3g

130. Marinated Cajun Beef

Servings: 2
Cooking Time: 20 Minutes
Ingredients:

- 1/3 cup beef broth
- 2 tablespoons Cajun seasoning, crushed
- 1/2 teaspoon garlic powder
- 3/4 pound beef tenderloins
- ½ tablespoon pear cider vinegar
- 1/3 teaspoon cayenne pepper
- 1 ½ tablespoon olive oil
- 1/2 teaspoon freshly ground black pepper
- 1 teaspoon salt

Directions:
1. Firstly, coat the beef tenderloins with salt, cayenne pepper, and black pepper.
2. Mix the remaining items in a medium-sized bowl; let the meat marinate for 40 minutes in this mixture.
3. Roast the beef for about 22 minutes at 385 degrees F, turning it halfway through the cooking time.
- **Nutrition Info:** 483 Calories; 23g Fat; 5g Carbs; 53g Protein; 6g Sugars; 4g Fiber

131. Coconut-crusted Haddock With Curried Pumpkin Seeds

Servings: 4
Cooking Time: 10 Minutes
Ingredients:
- 2 teaspoons canola oil
- 2 teaspoons honey
- 1 teaspoon curry powder
- 1/4 teaspoon ground cinnamon
- 1 teaspoon salt
- 1 cup pumpkin seeds
- 1-1/2 pounds haddock or cod filets
- 1/2 cup roughly grated unsweetened coconut
- 3/4 cups panko-style bread crumbs
- 2 tablespoons butter, melted
- 3 tablespoons apricot fruit spread
- 1 tablespoon lime juice

Directions:
1. Start by preheating toaster oven to 350°F.
2. In a medium bowl, mix honey, oil, curry powder, 1/2 teaspoon salt, and cinnamon.
3. Add pumpkin seeds to the bowl and toss to coat, then lay flat on a baking sheet.
4. Toast for 14 minutes, then transfer to a bowl to cool.
5. Increase the oven temperature to 450°F.
6. Brush a baking sheet with oil and lay filets flat.
7. In another medium mixing bowl, mix together bread crumbs, butter, and remaining salt.
8. In a small bowl mash together apricot spread and lime juice.
9. Brush each filet with apricot mixture, then press bread crumb mixture onto each piece.
10. Bake for 10 minutes.
11. Transfer to a plate and top with pumpkin seeds to serve.
- **Nutrition Info:** Calories: 273, Sodium: 491 mg, Dietary Fiber: 6.1 g, Total Fat: 8.4 g, Total Carbs: 47.3 g, Protein: 7.0 g.

132. Easy Air Fryed Roasted Asparagus

Servings: 4
Cooking Time: 10 Minutes
Ingredients:
- 1 bunch fresh asparagus
- 1 ½ tsp herbs de provence
- Fresh lemon wedge (optional)
- 1 tablespoon olive oil or cooking spray
- Salt and pepper to taste

Directions:
1. Wash asparagus and trim off hard ends
2. Drizzle asparagus with olive oil and add seasonings
3. Place asparagus in air fryer and cook on 360F for 6 to 10 minutes
4. Drizzle squeezed lemon over roasted asparagus.
- **Nutrition Info:** Calories 46 protein 2g fat 3g net carbs 1g

133. Creamy Breaded Shrimp

Servings: 3
Cooking Time: 20 Minutes
Ingredients:
- ¼ cup all-purpose flour
- 1 cup panko breadcrumbs
- 1 pound shrimp, peeled and deveined
- ½ cup mayonnaise
- ¼ cup sweet chili sauce
- 1 tablespoon Sriracha sauce

Directions:

1. Preheat the Air fryer to 400-degree F and grease an Air fryer basket.
2. Place flour in a shallow bowl and mix the mayonnaise, chili sauce, and Sriracha sauce in another bowl.
3. Place the breadcrumbs in a third bowl.
4. Coat each shrimp with the flour, dip into mayonnaise mixture and finally, dredge in the breadcrumbs.
5. Arrange half of the coated shrimps into the Air fryer basket and cook for about 10 minutes.
6. Dish out the coated shrimps onto serving plates and repeat with the remaining mixture.
- **Nutrition Info:** Calories: 540, Fat: 18.2g, Carbohydrates: 33.1g, Sugar: 10.6g, Protein: 36.8g, Sodium: 813mg

134. Chinese-style Spicy And Herby Beef

Servings: 4
Cooking Time: 20 Minutes
Ingredients:
- 1 pound flank steak, cut into small pieces
- 1 teaspoon fresh sage leaves, minced
- 1/3 cup olive oil
- 3 teaspoons sesame oil
- 3 tablespoons Shaoxing wine
- 2 tablespoons tamari
- 1 teaspoon hot sauce
- 1/8 teaspoon xanthum gum
- 1 teaspoon seasoned salt
- 3 cloves garlic, minced
- 1 teaspoon fresh rosemary leaves, finely minced
- 1/2 teaspoon freshly cracked black pepper

Directions:
1. Warm the oil in a sauté pan over a moderate heat. Now, sauté the garlic until just tender and fragrant.
2. Now, add the remaining ingredients. Toss to coat well.
3. Then, roast for about 18 minutes at 345 degrees F. Check doneness and serve warm.
- **Nutrition Info:** 354 Calories; 24g Fat; 8g Carbs; 21g Protein; 3g Sugars; 3g Fiber

135. Lemongrass Pork Chops

Servings: 3
Cooking Time: 2 Hrs 20 Minutes
Ingredients:
- 3 slices pork chops
- 2 garlic cloves, minced
- 1 ½ tbsp sugar
- 4 stalks lemongrass, trimmed and chopped
- 2 shallots, chopped
- 2 tbsp olive oil
- 1 ¼ tsp soy sauce
- 1 ¼ tsp fish sauce
- 1 ½ tsp black pepper

Directions:
1. In a bowl, add the garlic, sugar, lemongrass, shallots, olive oil, soy sauce, fish sauce, and black pepper; mix well. Add the pork chops, coat them with the mixture and allow to marinate for around 2 hours to get nice and savory.
2. Preheat the Air Fryer to 400 F. Cooking in 2 to 3 batches, remove and shake each pork chop from the marinade and place it in the fryer basket. Cook it for 7 minutes. Turn the pork chops with kitchen tongs and cook further for 5 minutes. Remove the chops and serve with a side of sautéed asparagus.
- **Nutrition Info:** 346 Calories; 11g Fat; 4g Carbs; 32g Protein; 1g Sugars; 1g Fiber

136. Broccoli With Olives

Servings: 4
Cooking Time: 19 Minutes
Ingredients:
- 2 pounds broccoli, stemmed and cut into 1-inch florets
- 1/3 cup Kalamata olives, halved and pitted
- ¼ cup Parmesan cheese, grated
- 2 tablespoons olive oil
- Salt and ground black pepper, as required
- 2 teaspoons fresh lemon zest, grated

Directions:
1. Preheat the Air fryer to 400 ºF and grease an Air fryer basket.
2. Boil the broccoli for about 4 minutes and drain well.

3. Mix broccoli, oil, salt, and black pepper in a bowl and toss to coat well.
4. Arrange broccoli into the Air fryer basket and cook for about 15 minutes.
5. Stir in the olives, lemon zest and cheese and dish out to serve.
- **Nutrition Info:** Calories: 169, Fat: 10.2g, Carbohydrates: 16g, Sugar: 3.9g, Protein: 8.5g, Sodium: 254mg

137. Artichoke Spinach Casserole

Servings: 4
Cooking Time: 20 Minutes
Ingredients:
- ⅓ cup full-fat mayonnaise
- oz. full-fat cream cheese; softened.
- ¼ cup diced yellow onion
- ⅓ cup full-fat sour cream.
- ¼ cup chopped pickled jalapeños.
- 2 cups fresh spinach; chopped
- 2 cups cauliflower florets; chopped
- 1 cup artichoke hearts; chopped
- 1 tbsp. salted butter; melted.

Directions:
1. Take a large bowl, mix butter, onion, cream cheese, mayonnaise and sour cream. Fold in jalapeños, spinach, cauliflower and artichokes.
2. Pour the mixture into a 4-cup round baking dish. Cover with foil and place into the air fryer basket
3. Adjust the temperature to 370 Degrees F and set the timer for 15 minutes. In the last 2 minutes of cooking, remove the foil to brown the top. Serve warm.
- **Nutrition Info:** Calories: 423; Protein: 7g; Fiber: 3g; Fat: 33g; Carbs: 11g

138. Beef, Mushrooms And Noodles Dish

Servings: 5
Cooking Time: 35 Minutes
Ingredients:
- 1½ pounds beef steak
- 1 package egg noodles, cooked
- 1 ounce dry onion soup mix
- 1 can (15 oz cream mushroom soup
- 2 cups mushrooms, sliced
- 1 whole onion, chopped
- ½ cup beef broth
- 3 garlic cloves, minced?

Directions:
1. Preheat your Air Fryer to 360 F. Drizzle onion soup mix all over the meat. In a mixing bowl, mix the sauce, garlic cloves, beef broth, chopped onion, sliced mushrooms and mushroom soup. Top the meat with the prepared sauce mixture. Place the prepared meat in the air fryer's cooking basket and cook for 25 minutes. Serve with cooked egg noodles.
- **Nutrition Info:** 346 Calories; 11g Fat; 4g Carbs; 32g Protein; 1g Sugars; 1g Fiber

139. Rice And Tuna Puff

Servings: 6
Cooking Time: 60 Minutes
Ingredients:
- 2/3 cup uncooked white rice
- 1 1/3 cups water
- 1/3 cup butter
- 1/4 cup all-purpose flour
- 1 teaspoon salt
- 1/4 teaspoon ground black pepper
- 1 1/2 cups milk
- 2 egg yolks
- 1 (12 ounces) can tuna, undrained
- 2 tablespoons grated onion
- 1 tablespoon lemon juice
- 2 egg whites

Directions:
1. In a saucepan, bring water to a boil. Stir in rice, cover, and cook on low heat until liquid is fully absorbed, around 20 minutes.
2. In another saucepan over medium heat, melt butter. Stir in pepper, salt, and flour. Cook for 2 minutes, whisking constantly and slowly adding milk. Continue cooking and stirring until thickened.
3. In a medium bowl, whisk egg yolks. Slowly whisk in half of the thickened milk mixture. Add to a pan of remaining milk and continue cooking and stirring for 2 more minutes. Stir in lemon juice, onion, tuna, and rice.
4. Place the instant pot air fryer lid on, lightly grease baking pan of the instant pot with

cooking spray. And transfer rice mixture into it.
5. Beat egg whites until stiff peak forms. Slowly fold into rice mixture.
6. Cover pan with foil, place the baking pan in the instant pot and close the air fryer lid.
7. Cook at 360 ºF for 20 minutes.
8. Cook for 15 minutes at 390 ºF until tops are lightly browned and the middle has set.
9. Serve and enjoy.
- **Nutrition Info:** Calories: 302; Carbs: 24.1g; Protein: 20.6g; Fat: 13.6g

140. Creole Beef Meatloaf

Servings: 6
Cooking Time: 15 Minutes
Ingredients:
- 1 lb. ground beef
- 1/2 tablespoon butter
- 1 red bell pepper diced
- 1/3 cup red onion diced
- 1/3 cup cilantro diced
- 1/3 cup zucchini diced
- 1 tablespoon creole seasoning
- 1/2 teaspoon turmeric
- 1/2 teaspoon cumin
- 1/2 teaspoon coriander
- 2 garlic cloves minced
- Salt and black pepper to taste

Directions:
1. Mix the beef minced with all the meatball ingredients in a bowl.
2. Make small meatballs out of this mixture and place them in the Air fryer basket.
3. Press "Power Button" of Air Fry Oven and turn the dial to select the "Air Fry" mode.
4. Press the Time button and again turn the dial to set the cooking time to 15 minutes.
5. Now push the Temp button and rotate the dial to set the temperature at 370 degrees F.
6. Once preheated, place the Air fryer basket in the oven and close its lid.
7. Slice and serve warm.
- **Nutrition Info:** Calories: 331 Cal Total Fat: 2.5 gSaturated Fat: 0.5 g Cholesterol: 35 mg Sodium: 595 mg Total Carbs: 69 g Fiber: 12.2 g Sugar: 12.5 g Protein: 26.7 g

141. Tex-mex Chicken Quesadillas

Servings: 4
Cooking Time: 10 Minutes
Ingredients:
- 2 green onions
- 2 cups shredded skinless rotisserie chicken meat
- 1-1/2 cups shredded Monterey Jack cheese
- 1 pickled jalapeño
- 1/4 cup fresh cilantro leaves
- 4 burrito-size flour tortillas
- 1/2 cup reduced-fat sour cream

Directions:
1. Start by preheating toaster oven to 425°F.
2. Thinly slice the green onions and break apart.
3. Mix together chicken, cheese, jalapeño, and onions in a bowl, then evenly divide mixture onto one half of each tortilla.
4. Fold opposite half over mixture and place quesadillas onto a baking sheet.
5. Bake for 10 minutes.
6. Cut in halves or quarters and serve with sour cream.
- **Nutrition Info:** Calories: 830, Sodium: 921 mg, Dietary Fiber: 1.8 g, Total Fat: 59.0 g, Total Carbs: 13.8 g, Protein: 60.8 g.

142. Broccoli Stuffed Peppers

Servings: 2
Cooking Time: 40 Minutes
Ingredients:
- 4 eggs
- 1/2 cup cheddar cheese, grated
- 2 bell peppers, cut in half and remove seeds 1/2 tsp garlic powder
- 1 tsp dried thyme
- 1/4 cup feta cheese, crumbled 1/2 cup broccoli, cooked
- 1/4 tsp pepper 1/2 tsp salt

Directions:
1. Preheat the air fryer to 325 F.
2. Stuff feta and broccoli into the bell peppers halved.
3. Beat egg in a bowl with seasoning and pour egg mixture into the pepper halved over feta and broccoli.

4. Place bell pepper halved into the air fryer basket and cook for 35-40 minutes.
5. Top with grated cheddar cheese and cook until cheese melted.
6. Serve and enjoy.
- **Nutrition Info:** Calories 340 Fat 22 g Carbohydrates 12 g Sugar 8.2 g Protein 22 g Cholesterol 374 mg

143. Indian Meatballs With Lamb

Servings: 8
Cooking Time: 14 Minutes
Ingredients:
- 1 garlic clove
- 1 tablespoon butter
- 4 oz chive stems
- ¼ tablespoon turmeric
- 1/3 teaspoon cayenne pepper
- 1 teaspoon ground coriander
- ¼ teaspoon bay leaf
- 1 teaspoon salt
- 1-pound ground lamb
- 1 egg
- 1 teaspoon ground black pepper

Directions:
1. Peel the garlic clove and mince it
2. Combine the minced garlic with the ground lamb.
3. Then sprinkle the meat mixture with the turmeric, cayenne pepper, ground coriander, bay leaf, salt, and ground black pepper.
4. Beat the egg in the forcemeat.
5. Then grate the chives and add them in the lamb forcemeat too.
6. Mix it up to make the smooth mass.
7. Then preheat the air fryer to 400 F.
8. Put the butter in the air fryer basket tray and melt it.
9. Then make the meatballs from the lamb mixture and place them in the air fryer basket tray.
10. Cook the dish for 14 minutes.
11. Stir the meatballs twice during the cooking.
12. Serve the cooked meatballs immediately.
13. Enjoy!
- **Nutrition Info:** calories 134, fat 6.2, fiber 0.4, carbs 1.8, protein 16.9

144. Pesto & White Wine Salmon

Servings: 4
Cooking Time: 10 Minutes
Ingredients:
- 1-1/4 pounds salmon filet
- 2 tablespoons white wine
- 2 tablespoons pesto
- 1 lemon

Directions:
1. Cut the salmon into 4 pieces and place on a greased baking sheet.
2. Slice the lemon into quarters and squeeze 1 quarter over each piece of salmon.
3. Drizzle wine over salmon and set aside to marinate while preheating the toaster oven on broil.
4. Spread pesto over each piece of salmon.
5. Broil for at least 10 minutes, or until the fish is cooked to desired doneness and the pesto is browned.
- **Nutrition Info:** Calories: 236, Sodium: 111 mg, Dietary Fiber: 0.9 g, Total Fat: 12.1 g, Total Carbs: 3.3 g, Protein: 28.6 g.

145. Air Fryer Buffalo Mushroom Poppers

Servings: 8
Cooking Time: 50 Minutes
Ingredients:
- 1 pound fresh whole button mushrooms
- 1/2 teaspoon kosher salt
- 3 tablespoons 1/3-less-fat cream cheese,
- 1/4 cup all-purpose flour
- Softened 1 jalapeño chile, seeded and minced
- Cooking spray
- 1/4 teaspoon black pepper
- 1 cup panko breadcrumbs
- 2 large eggs, lightly beaten
- 1/4 cup buffalo-style hot sauce
- 2 tablespoons chopped fresh chives
- 1/2 cup low-fat buttermilk
- 1/2 cup plain fat-free yogurt
- 2 ounces blue cheese, crumbled (about 1/2 cup)
- 3 tablespoons apple cider vinegar

Directions:

1. Remove stems from mushroom caps, chop stems and set caps aside. Stir together chopped mushroom stems, cream cheese, jalapeño, salt, and pepper. Stuff about 1 teaspoon of the mixture into each mushroom cap, rounding the filling to form a smooth ball.
2. Place panko in a bowl, place flour in a second bowl, and eggs in a third Coat mushrooms in flour, dip in egg mixture, and dredge in panko, pressing to adhere. Spray mushrooms well with cooking spray.
3. Place half of the mushrooms in air fryer basket, and cook for 20 minutes at 350°F. Transfer cooked mushrooms to a large bowl. Drizzle buffalo sauce over mushrooms; toss to coat then sprinkle with chives.
4. Stir buttermilk, yogurt, blue cheese, and cider vinegar in a small bowl. Serve mushroom poppers with blue cheese sauce.
- **Nutrition Info:** Calories 133 Fat 4g Saturated fat 2g Unsaturated fat 2g Protein 7g Carbohydrate 16g Fiber 1g Sugars 3g Sodium 485mg Calcium 10% DV Potassium 7% DV

146. Roasted Garlic Zucchini Rolls

Servings: 4
Cooking Time: 20 Minutes
Ingredients:
- 2 medium zucchinis
- ½ cup full-fat ricotta cheese
- ¼ white onion; peeled. And diced
- 2 cups spinach; chopped
- ¼ cup heavy cream
- ½ cup sliced baby portobello mushrooms
- ¾ cup shredded mozzarella cheese, divided.
- 2 tbsp. unsalted butter.
- 2 tbsp. vegetable broth.
- ½ tsp. finely minced roasted garlic
- ¼ tsp. dried oregano.
- ⅛ tsp. xanthan gum
- ¼ tsp. salt
- ½ tsp. garlic powder.

Directions:
1. Using a mandoline or sharp knife, slice zucchini into long strips lengthwise. Place strips between paper towels to absorb moisture. Set aside
2. In a medium saucepan over medium heat, melt butter. Add onion and sauté until fragrant. Add garlic and sauté 30 seconds.
3. Pour in heavy cream, broth and xanthan gum. Turn off heat and whisk mixture until it begins to thicken, about 3 minutes.
4. Take a medium bowl, add ricotta, salt, garlic powder and oregano and mix well. Fold in spinach, mushrooms and ½ cup mozzarella
5. Pour half of the sauce into a 6-inch round baking pan. To assemble the rolls, place two strips of zucchini on a work surface. Spoon 2 tbsp. of ricotta mixture onto the slices and roll up. Place seam side down on top of sauce. Repeat with remaining ingredients
6. Pour remaining sauce over the rolls and sprinkle with remaining mozzarella. Cover with foil and place into the air fryer basket. Adjust the temperature to 350 Degrees F and set the timer for 20 minutes. In the last 5 minutes, remove the foil to brown the cheese. Serve immediately.
- **Nutrition Info:** Calories: 245; Protein: 15g; Fiber: 8g; Fat: 19g; Carbs: 1g

147. Creamy Tuna Cakes

Servings: 4
Cooking Time: 15 Minutes
Ingredients:
- 2: 6-ouncescans tuna, drained
- 1½ tablespoon almond flour
- 1½ tablespoons mayonnaise
- 1 tablespoon fresh lemon juice
- 1 teaspoon dried dill
- 1 teaspoon garlic powder
- ½ teaspoon onion powder
- Pinch of salt and ground black pepper

Directions:
1. Preheat the Air fryer to 400-degree F and grease an Air fryer basket.
2. Mix the tuna, mayonnaise, almond flour, lemon juice, dill, and spices in a large bowl.
3. Make 4 equal-sized patties from the mixture and arrange in the Air fryer basket.
4. Cook for about 10 minutes and flip the sides.

5. Cook for 5 more minutes and dish out the tuna cakes in serving plates to serve warm.
- **Nutrition Info:** Calories: 200, Fat: 10.1g, Carbohydrates: 2.9g, Sugar: 0.8g, Protein: 23.4g, Sodium: 122mg

148. Traditional English Fish And Chips

Servings: 4
Cooking Time: 17 Minutes
Ingredients:
- 1 3/4 pounds potatoes
- 4 tablespoons olive oil
- 1-1/4 teaspoons kosher salt
- 1-1/4 teaspoons black pepper
- 8 sprigs fresh thyme
- 4 (6-ounce) pieces cod
- 1 lemon
- 1 clove garlic
- 2 tablespoons capers

Directions:
1. Start by preheating toaster oven to 450°F.
2. Cut potatoes into 1-inch chunks.
3. Place potatoes, 2 tablespoons oil, salt, and thyme in a baking tray and toss to combine.
4. Spread in a flat layer and bake for 30 minutes.
5. Wrap mixture in foil to keep warm.
6. Wipe tray with a paper towel and then lay cod in the tray.
7. Slice the lemon and top cod with lemon, salt, pepper, and thyme.
8. Drizzle rest of the oil over the cod and bake for 12 minutes.
9. Place cod and potatoes on separate pans and bake together for an additional 5 minutes.
10. Combine and serve.
- **Nutrition Info:** Calories: 442, Sodium: 1002 mg, Dietary Fiber: 5.4 g, Total Fat: 15.8 g, Total Carbs: 32.7 g, Protein: 42.5 g.

149. Pork Chops With Chicory Treviso

Servings: 2
Cooking Time: 0-15;
Ingredients:
- 4 pork chops
- 40g butter
- Flour to taste
- 1 chicory stalk
- Salt to taste

Directions:
1. Cut the chicory into small pieces. Place the butter and chicory in pieces on the basket of the air fryer previously preheated at 1800C and brown for 2 min.
2. Add the previously floured and salted pork slices (directly over the chicory), simmer for 6 minutes turning them over after 3 minutes.
3. Remove the slices and place them on a serving plate, covering them with the rest of the red chicory juice collected at the bottom of the basket.
- **Nutrition Info:** Calories 504, Fat 33, Carbohydrates 0g, Sugars 0g, Protein 42g, Cholesterol 130mg

150. Grilled Tasty Scallops

Servings: 2
Cooking Time: 10 Minutes
Ingredients:
- 1 pound sea scallops, cleaned and patted dry
- Salt and pepper to taste
- 3 dried chilies
- 2 tablespoon dried thyme
- 1 tablespoon dried oregano
- 1 tablespoon ground coriander
- 1 tablespoon ground fennel
- 2 teaspoons chipotle pepper

Directions:
1. Place the instant pot air fryer lid on and preheat the instant pot at 390 degrees F.
2. Place the grill pan accessory in the instant pot.
3. Mix all ingredients in a bowl.
4. Dump the scallops on the grill pan, close the air fryer lid and cook for 10 minutes.
- **Nutrition Info:** Calories:291 ; Carbs: 20.7g; Protein: 48.6g; Fat: 2.5g

151. Cheesy Shrimp

Servings: 4
Cooking Time: 20 Minutes
Ingredients:
- 2/3 cup Parmesan cheese, grated

- 2 pounds shrimp, peeled and deveined
- 4 garlic cloves, minced
- 2 tablespoons olive oil
- 1 teaspoon dried basil
- ½ teaspoon dried oregano
- 1 teaspoon onion powder
- ½ teaspoon red pepper flakes, crushed
- Ground black pepper, as required
- 2 tablespoons fresh lemon juice

Directions:
1. Preheat the Air fryer to 350 degree F and grease an Air fryer basket.
2. Mix Parmesan cheese, garlic, olive oil, herbs, and spices in a large bowl.
3. Arrange half of the shrimp into the Air fryer basket in a single layer and cook for about 10 minutes.
4. Dish out the shrimps onto serving plates and drizzle with lemon juice to serve hot.
- **Nutrition Info:** Calories: 386, Fat: 14.2g, Carbohydrates: 5.3g, Sugar: 0.4g, Protein: 57.3g, Sodium: 670mg

152. Morning Ham And Cheese Sandwich

Servings: 4
Cooking Time: 15 Minutes
Ingredients:
- 8 slices whole wheat bread
- 4 slices lean pork ham
- 4 slices cheese
- 8 slices tomato

Directions:
1. Preheat your air fryer to 360 f. Lay four slices of bread on a flat surface. Spread the slices with cheese, tomato, turkey and ham. Cover with the remaining slices to form sandwiches. Add the sandwiches to the air fryer cooking basket and cook for 10 minutes.
- **Nutrition Info:** Calories: 361 Cal Total Fat: 16.7 g Saturated Fat: 0 g Cholesterol: 0 mg Sodium: 1320 mg Total Carbs: 32.5 g Fiber: 2.3 g Sugar: 5.13 g Protein: 19.3 g

153. Coco Mug Cake

Servings: 1
Cooking Time: 20 Minutes
Ingredients:

- 1 large egg.
- 2 tbsp. granular erythritol.
- 2 tbsp. coconut flour.
- 2 tbsp. heavy whipping cream.
- ¼ tsp. baking powder.
- ¼ tsp. vanilla extract.

Directions:
1. In a 4-inch ramekin, whisk egg, then add remaining ingredients. Stir until smooth. Place into the air fryer basket.
2. Adjust the temperature to 300 Degrees F and set the timer for 25 minutes.
3. When done a toothpick should come out clean. Enjoy right out of the ramekin with a spoon. Serve warm.
- **Nutrition Info:** Calories: 237; Protein: 9g; Fiber: 0g; Fat: 14g; Carbs: 47g

154. Cinnamon Pork Rinds

Servings: 2
Cooking Time: 20 Minutes
Ingredients:
- 2 oz. pork rinds
- ¼ cup powdered erythritol
- 2 tbsp. unsalted butter; melted.
- ½ tsp. ground cinnamon.

Directions:
1. Take a large bowl, toss pork rinds and butter. Sprinkle with cinnamon and erythritol, then toss to evenly coat.
2. Place pork rinds into the air fryer basket. Adjust the temperature to 400 Degrees F and set the timer for 5 minutes. Serve immediately.
- **Nutrition Info:** Calories: 264; Protein: 13g; Fiber: 4g; Fat: 28g; Carbs: 15g

155. Smoked Ham With Pears

Servings: 2
Cooking Time: 30 Minutes
Ingredients:
- 15 oz pears, halved
- 8 pound smoked ham
- 1 ½ cups brown sugar
- ¾ tbsp allspice
- 1 tbsp apple cider vinegar
- 1 tsp black pepper
- 1 tsp vanilla extract

Directions:
1. Preheat your air fryer to 330 f. In a bowl, mix pears, brown sugar, cider vinegar, vanilla extract, pepper, and allspice. Place the mixture in a frying pan and fry for 2-3 minutes. Pour the mixture over ham. Add the ham to the air fryer cooking basket and cook for 15 minutes. Serve ham with hot sauce, to enjoy!
- **Nutrition Info:** Calories: 550 Cal Total Fat: 29 g Saturated Fat: 0 g Cholesterol: 0 mg Sodium: 0 mg Total Carbs: 46 g Fiber: 0 g Sugar: 0 g Protein: 28 g

156.Vegetable Cane

Servings: 4
Cooking Time: More Than 60 Minutes;
Ingredients:
- 2 calf legs
- 4 carrots
- 4 medium potatoes
- 1 clove garlic
- 300ml Broth
- Leave to taste
- Pepper to taste

Directions:
1. Place the ears, garlic, and half of the broth in the greased basket.
2. Set the temperature to 1800C.
3. Cook the stems for 40 minutes, turning them in the middle of cooking.
4. Add the vegetables in pieces, salt, pepper, pour the rest of the broth and cook for another 50 minutes (time may vary depending on the size of the hocks).
5. Mix the vegetables and the ears 2 to 3 times during cooking.
- **Nutrition Info:** Calories 7.9, Fat 0.49g, Carbohydrate 0.77g, Sugar 0.49g, Protein 0.08mg, Cholesterol 0mg

MEAT RECIPES

157. Cracker Apple Chicken

Servings: 2
Cooking Time: 45 Minutes
Ingredients:
- 2 chicken breasts, skinless and boneless
- 1 apple, sliced
- 12 Ritz cracker, crushed
- 10 oz can condensed cheddar cheese soup
- Pepper
- Salt

Directions:
1. Fit the Kalorik Maxx oven with the rack in position
2. Season chicken with pepper and salt and place into the baking dish.
3. Arrange sliced apple on top of chicken.
4. Sprinkle crushed crackers on top.
5. Set to bake at 350 F for 50 minutes. After 5 minutes place the baking dish in the preheated oven.
6. Pour cheddar cheese soup on top and serve.
- **Nutrition Info:** Calories 924 Fat 38.2 g Carbohydrates 87 g Sugar 21.4 g Protein 51.8 g Cholesterol 136 mg

158. Beef Rolls With Pesto & Spinach

Servings: 4
Cooking Time: 30 Minutes
Ingredients:
- 2 pounds beef steaks, sliced
- Salt and black pepper to taste
- 3 tbsp pesto
- 6 slices mozzarella cheese
- ¾ cup spinach, chopped
- 3 oz bell pepper, deseeded and sliced

Directions:
1. Top the meat with pesto, mozzarella cheese, spinach, and bell pepper. Roll up the slices and secure using a toothpick. Season with salt and pepper. Place the slices in the basket and fit in the baking tray; cook for 15 minutes on Air Fry function at 400 F, turning once. Serve immediately!

159. Teriyaki Chicken Thighs With Lemony Snow Peas

Servings: 4
Cooking Time: 34 Minutes
Ingredients:
- ¼ cup chicken broth
- ½ teaspoon grated fresh ginger
- ⅛ teaspoon red pepper flakes
- 1½ tablespoons soy sauce
- 4 (5-ounce / 142-g) bone-in chicken thighs, trimmed
- 1 tablespoon mirin
- ½ teaspoon cornstarch
- 1 tablespoon sugar
- 6 ounces (170 g) snow peas, strings removed
- ⅛ teaspoon lemon zest
- 1 garlic clove, minced
- ¼ teaspoon salt
- Ground black pepper, to taste
- ½ teaspoon lemon juice

Directions:
1. Combine the broth, ginger, pepper flakes, and soy sauce in a large bowl. Stir to mix well.
2. Pierce 10 to 15 holes into the chicken skin. Put the chicken in the broth mixture and toss to coat well. Let sit for 10 minutes to marinate.
3. Transfer the marinated chicken on a plate and pat dry with paper towels.
4. Scoop 2 tablespoons of marinade in a microwave-safe bowl and combine with mirin, cornstarch and sugar. Stir to mix well. Microwave for 1 minute or until frothy and has a thick consistency. Set aside.
5. Arrange the chicken in the air fryer basket, skin side up.
6. Put the air fryer basket on the baking pan and slide into Rack Position 2, select Air Fry, set temperature to 400ºF (205ºC) and set time to 25 minutes.
7. Flip the chicken halfway through.
8. When cooking is complete, brush the chicken skin with marinade mixture. Air fry

the chicken for 5 more minutes or until glazed.
9. Remove the chicken from the oven. Allow the chicken to cool for 10 minutes.
10. Meanwhile, combine the snow peas, lemon zest, garlic, salt, and ground black pepper in a small bowl. Toss to coat well.
11. Transfer the snow peas in the basket.
12. Put the air fryer basket on the baking pan and slide into Rack Position 2, select Air Fry, set temperature to 400ºF (205ºC) and set time to 3 minutes.
13. When cooking is complete, the peas should be soft.
14. Remove the peas from the oven and toss with lemon juice.
15. Serve the chicken with lemony snow peas.

160. Lemon Mustard Chicken

Servings: 4
Cooking Time: 20 Minutes
Ingredients:
- 1 lbs chicken tenders
- 1 garlic clove, minced
- 1/2 oz fresh lemon juice
- 1/2 tsp pepper
- 2 tbsp fresh tarragon, chopped
- 1/2 cup whole grain mustard
- 1/2 tsp paprika
- 1/4 tsp kosher salt

Directions:
1. Fit the Kalorik Maxx oven with the rack in position
2. Add all ingredients except chicken to the large bowl and mix well.
3. Add chicken to the bowl and stir until well coated.
4. Place chicken in a baking dish.
5. Set to bake at 425 F for 25 minutes. After 5 minutes place the baking dish in the preheated oven.
6. Serve and enjoy.
- **Nutrition Info:** Calories 242 Fat 9.5 g Carbohydrates 3.1 g Sugar 0.1 g Protein 33.2 g Cholesterol 101 mg

161. Air Fried London Broil

Servings: 6
Cooking Time: 25 Minutes
Ingredients:
- 2 tablespoons Worcestershire sauce
- 2 tablespoons minced onion
- ¼ cup honey
- ²/₃ cup ketchup
- 2 tablespoons apple cider vinegar
- ½ teaspoon paprika
- ¼ cup olive oil
- 1 teaspoon salt
- 1 teaspoon freshly ground black pepper
- 2 pounds (907 g) London broil, top round (about 1-inch thick)

Directions:
1. Combine all the ingredients, except for the London broil, in a large bowl. Stir to mix well.
2. Pierce the meat with a fork generously on both sides, then dunk the meat in the mixture and press to coat well.
3. Wrap the bowl in plastic and refrigerate to marinate for at least 8 hours.
4. Discard the marinade and transfer the London broil to the basket.
5. Put the air fryer basket on the baking pan and slide into Rack Position 2, select Air Fry, set temperature to 400ºF (205ºC) and set time to 25 minutes.
6. Flip the meat halfway through the cooking time.
7. When cooking is complete, the meat should be well browned.
8. Transfer the cooked London broil on a plate and allow to cool for 5 minutes before slicing to serve.

162. Citrus Carnitas

Servings: 6
Cooking Time: 25 Minutes
Ingredients:
- 2½ pounds (1.1 kg) boneless country-style pork ribs, cut into 2-inch pieces
- 3 tablespoons olive brine
- 1 tablespoon minced fresh oregano leaves
- ¹/₃ cup orange juice
- 1 teaspoon ground cumin
- 1 tablespoon minced garlic
- 1 teaspoon salt

- 1 teaspoon ground black pepper
- Cooking spray

Directions:
1. Combine all the ingredients in a large bowl. Toss to coat the pork ribs well. Wrap the bowl in plastic and refrigerate for at least an hour to marinate.
2. Spritz the air fryer basket with cooking spray.
3. Arrange the marinated pork ribs in the pan and spritz with cooking spray.
4. Put the air fryer basket on the baking pan and slide into Rack Position 2, select Air Fry, set temperature to 400ºF (205ºC) and set time to 25 minutes.
5. Flip the ribs halfway through.
6. When cooking is complete, the ribs should be well browned.
7. Serve immediately.

163. Chicken & Cheese Enchilada

Servings: 4
Cooking Time: 35 Minutes
Ingredients:
- 1 lb chicken breasts, chopped
- 2 cups cheddar cheese, grated
- ½ cup salsa
- 1 can green chilies, chopped
- 12 flour tortillas
- 2 cups enchilada sauce

Directions:
1. In a bowl, mix salsa and enchilada sauce. Toss in the chopped chicken to coat. Place the chicken on the tortillas and roll; top with cheese. Place the prepared tortillas in a baking tray and press Start. Cook for 25-30 minutes at 400 F on Bake function. Serve with guacamole and hot dips!

164. Spice-coated Steaks With Cucumber And Snap Pea Salad

Servings: 4
Cooking Time: 15 Minutes
Ingredients:
- 1 (1½-pound / 680-g) boneless top sirloin steak, trimmed and halved crosswise
- 1½ teaspoons chili powder
- 1½ teaspoons ground cumin
- ¾ teaspoon ground coriander
- ⅛ teaspoon cayenne pepper
- ⅛ teaspoon ground cinnamon
- 1¼ teaspoons plus ⅛ teaspoon salt, divided
- ½ teaspoon plus ⅛ teaspoon ground black pepper, divided
- 1 teaspoon plus 1½ tablespoons extra-virgin olive oil, divided
- 3 tablespoons mayonnaise
- 1½ tablespoons white wine vinegar
- 1 tablespoon minced fresh dill
- 1 small garlic clove, minced
- 8 ounces (227 g) sugar snap peas, strings removed and cut in half on bias
- ½ English cucumber, halved lengthwise and sliced thin
- 2 radishes, trimmed, halved and sliced thin
- 2 cups baby arugula

Directions:
1. In a bowl, mix chili powder, cumin, coriander, cayenne pepper, cinnamon, 1¼ teaspoons salt and ½ teaspoon pepper until well combined.
2. Add the steaks to another bowl and pat dry with paper towels. Brush with 1 teaspoon oil and transfer to the bowl of spice mixture. Roll over to coat thoroughly.
3. Arrange the coated steaks in the basket, spaced evenly apart.
4. Put the air fryer basket on the baking pan and slide into Rack Position 2, select Air Fry, set temperature to 400ºF (205ºC) and set time to 15 minutes.
5. Flip the steak halfway through to ensure even cooking.
6. When cooking is complete, an instant-read thermometer inserted in the thickest part of the meat should register at least 145ºF (63ºC).
7. Transfer the steaks to a clean work surface and wrap with aluminum foil. Let stand while preparing salad.
8. Make the salad: In a large bowl, stir together 1½ tablespoons olive oil, mayonnaise, vinegar, dill, garlic, ⅛ teaspoon salt, and ⅛ teaspoon pepper. Add snap peas, cucumber, radishes and arugula. Toss to blend well.

9. Slice the steaks and serve with the salad.

165. Tuscan Air Fried Veal Loin

Servings: 3 Veal Chops
Cooking Time: 12 Minutes
Ingredients:
- 1½ teaspoons crushed fennel seeds
- 1 tablespoon minced fresh rosemary leaves
- 1 tablespoon minced garlic
- 1½ teaspoons lemon zest
- 1½ teaspoons salt
- ½ teaspoon red pepper flakes
- 2 tablespoons olive oil
- 3 (10-ounce / 284-g) bone-in veal loin, about ½ inch thick

Directions:
1. Combine all the ingredients, except for the veal loin, in a large bowl. Stir to mix well.
2. Dunk the loin in the mixture and press to submerge. Wrap the bowl in plastic and refrigerate for at least an hour to marinate.
3. Arrange the veal loin in the basket.
4. Put the air fryer basket on the baking pan and slide into Rack Position 2, select Air Fry, set temperature to 400ºF (205ºC) and set time to 12 minutes.
5. Flip the veal halfway through.
6. When cooking is complete, the internal temperature of the veal should reach at least 145ºF (63ºC) for medium rare.
7. Serve immediately.

166. Honey Bbq Lamb Chops

Servings: 6
Cooking Time: 10 Minutes
Ingredients:
- Nonstick cooking spray
- 2 tbsp. tomato sauce
- 2 tbsp. honey
- 1 tsp garlic, crushed
- 1 tsp green chili, diced fine
- 12 lamb loin chops or cutlets

Directions:
1. Place baking pan in position 2 of the oven. Lightly spray the fryer basket with cooking spray.
2. In a small bowl, whisk together tomato sauce, honey, garlic, and green chili.
3. Heat the oven to broil on 400°F for 15 minutes.
4. Brush both sides of lamb with sauce. Place in a single layer in the basket, you will need to cook them in batches.
5. After the oven preheats for 5 minutes, place basket on the baking pan. Cook 6-7 minutes, turning chops over halfway through cooking time. Serve immediately.
- **Nutrition Info:** Calories 372, Total Fat 6g, Saturated Fat 2g, Total Carbs 6g, Net Carbs 6g, Protein 17g, Sugar 6g, Fiber 0g, Sodium 91mg, Potassium 296mg, Phosphorus 161mg

167. Rosemary Turkey Scotch Eggs

Servings: 4
Cooking Time: 12 Minutes
Ingredients:
- 1 egg
- 1 cup panko bread crumbs
- ½ teaspoon rosemary
- 1 pound (454 g) ground turkey
- 4 hard-boiled eggs, peeled
- Salt and ground black pepper, to taste
- Cooking spray

Directions:
1. Spritz the air fryer basket with cooking spray.
2. Whisk the egg with salt in a bowl. Combine the bread crumbs with rosemary in a shallow dish.
3. Stir the ground turkey with salt and ground black pepper in a separate large bowl, then divide the ground turkey into four portions.
4. Wrap each hard-boiled egg with a portion of ground turkey. Dredge in the whisked egg, then roll over the breadcrumb mixture.
5. Place the wrapped eggs in the basket and spritz with cooking spray.
6. Put the air fryer basket on the baking pan and slide into Rack Position 2, select Air Fry, set temperature to 400ºF (205ºC) and set time to 12 minutes.
7. Flip the eggs halfway through.
8. When cooking is complete, the scotch eggs should be golden brown and crunchy.
9. Serve immediately.

168. Parmesan Cajun Pork Chops

Servings: 2
Cooking Time: 9 Minutes
Ingredients:
- 2 pork chops, boneless
- 1 tsp dried mixed herbs
- 1 tsp paprika
- 3 tbsp parmesan cheese, grated
- 1 tsp Cajun seasoning
- 1/3 cup almond flour

Directions:
1. Fit the Kalorik Maxx oven with the rack in position 2.
2. Line the air fryer basket with parchment paper.
3. In a shallow dish, mix parmesan cheese, almond flour, paprika, mixed herbs, and Cajun seasoning.
4. Spray pork chops with cooking spray and coat with parmesan cheese.
5. Place coated pork chops in the air fryer basket then place an air fryer basket in the baking pan.
6. Place a baking pan on the oven rack. Set to air fry at 350 F for 9 minutes.
7. Serve and enjoy.
- **Nutrition Info:** Calories 324 Fat 24.8 g Carbohydrates 2.2 g Sugar 0.3 g Protein 22.9 g Cholesterol 77 mg

169. Chicken Thighs With Radish Slaw

Servings: 4
Cooking Time: 27 Minutes
Ingredients:
- 4 bone-in, skin-on chicken thighs
- 1½ teaspoon kosher salt, divided
- 1 tablespoon smoked paprika
- ½ teaspoon granulated garlic
- ½ teaspoon dried oregano
- ¼ teaspoon freshly ground black pepper
- 3 cups shredded cabbage
- ½ small red onion, thinly sliced
- 4 large radishes, julienned
- 3 tablespoons red wine vinegar
- 2 tablespoons olive oil
- Cooking spray

Directions:
1. Salt the chicken thighs on both sides with 1 teaspoon of kosher salt. In a small bowl, combine the paprika, garlic, oregano, and black pepper. Sprinkle half this mixture over the skin sides of the thighs. Spritz the baking pan with cooking spray and place the thighs skin-side down in the pan. Sprinkle the remaining spice mixture over the other sides of the chicken pieces.
2. Slide the baking pan into Rack Position 2, select Roast, set temperature to 375ºF (190ºC), and set time to 27 minutes.
3. After 10 minutes, remove from the oven and turn over the chicken thighs. Return to the oven and continue cooking.
4. While the chicken cooks, place the cabbage, onion, and radishes in a large bowl. Sprinkle with the remaining kosher salt, vinegar, and olive oil. Toss to coat.
5. After another 9 to 10 minutes, remove from the oven and place the chicken thighs on a cutting board. Place the cabbage mixture in the pan and toss with the chicken fat and spices.
6. Spread the cabbage in an even layer on the pan and place the chicken on it, skin-side up. Return the pan to the oven and continue cooking. Roast for another 7 to 8 minutes.
7. When cooking is complete, the cabbage is just becoming tender. Remove from the oven. Taste and adjust the seasoning if necessary. Serve.

170. Barbecue Chicken And Coleslaw Tostadas

Servings: 4 Tostadas
Cooking Time: 10 Minutes
Ingredients:
- Coleslaw:
- ¼ cup sour cream
- ¼ small green cabbage, finely chopped
- ½ tablespoon white vinegar
- ½ teaspoon garlic powder
- ½ teaspoon salt
- ¼ teaspoon ground black pepper
- Tostadas:
- 2 cups pulled rotisserie chicken
- ½ cup barbecue sauce

- 4 corn tortillas
- ½ cup shredded Mozzarella cheese
- Cooking spray

Directions:
1. Make the Coleslaw:
2. Combine the ingredients for the coleslaw in a large bowl. Toss to mix well.
3. Refrigerate until ready to serve.
4. Make the Tostadas:
5. Spritz the air fryer basket with cooking spray.
6. Toss the chicken with barbecue sauce in a separate large bowl to combine well. Set aside.
7. Place one tortilla in the basket and spritz with cooking spray.
8. Put the air fryer basket on the baking pan and slide into Rack Position 2, select Air Fry, set temperature to 370ºF (188ºC) and set time to 10 minutes.
9. Flip the tortilla and spread the barbecue chicken and cheese over halfway through.
10. When cooking is complete, the tortilla should be browned and the cheese should be melted.
11. Serve the tostadas with coleslaw on top.

171. Cheesy Pepperoni And Chicken Pizza

Servings: 6
Cooking Time: 15 Minutes
Ingredients:
- 2 cups cooked chicken, cubed
- 1 cup pizza sauce
- 20 slices pepperoni
- ¼ cup grated Parmesan cheese
- 1 cup shredded Mozzarella cheese
- Cooking spray

Directions:
1. Spritz the baking pan with cooking spray.
2. Arrange the chicken cubes in the prepared baking pan, then top the cubes with pizza sauce and pepperoni. Stir to coat the cubes and pepperoni with sauce. Scatter the cheeses on top.
3. Put the air fryer basket on the baking pan and slide into Rack Position 2, select Air Fry, set temperature to 375ºF (190ºC) and set time to 15 minutes.
4. When cooking is complete, the pizza should be frothy and the cheeses should be melted.
5. Serve immediately.

172. Juicy Spicy Lemon Kebab

Servings: x
Cooking Time: x
Ingredients:
- 2 tsp. garam masala
- 4 tbsp. chopped coriander
- 3 tbsp. cream
- 2 tbsp. coriander powder
- 4 tbsp. fresh mint (chopped)
- 3 tbsp. chopped capsicum
- 2 lb. chicken breasts cubed
- 3 onions chopped
- 5 green chilies-roughly chopped
- 1 ½ tbsp. ginger paste
- 1 ½ tsp. garlic paste
- 1 ½ tsp. salt
- 3 tsp. lemon juice
- 2 tbsp. peanut flour
- 3 eggs

Directions:
1. Mix the dry ingredients in a bowl. Make the mixture into a smooth paste and coat the chicken cubes with the mixture. Beat the eggs in a bowl and add a little salt to them. Dip the cubes in the egg mixture and coat them with sesame seeds and leave them in the refrigerator for an hour. Pre heat the Kalorik Maxx oven at 290 Fahrenheit for around 5 minutes.
2. Place the kebabs in the basket and let them cook for another 25 minutes at the same temperature. Turn the kebabs over in between the cooking process to get a uniform cook. Serve the kebabs with mint sauce.

173. Beef Steak Oregano Fingers

Servings: x
Cooking Time: x
Ingredients:
- 1 lb. boneless beef steak cut into Oregano Fingers
- 2 cup dry breadcrumbs
- 4 tbsp. lemon juice

- 2 tsp. salt
- 1 tsp. pepper powder
- 1 tsp. red chili powder
- 6 tbsp. corn flour
- 4 eggs
- 2 tsp. oregano
- 2 tsp. red chili flakes
- 1 ½ tbsp. ginger-garlic paste

Directions:
1. Mix all the ingredients for the marinade and put the beef Oregano Fingers inside and let it rest overnight. Mix the breadcrumbs, oregano and red chili flakes well and place the marinated Oregano Fingers on this mixture. Cover it with plastic wrap and leave it till right before you serve to cook. Pre heat the Kalorik Maxx oven at 160 degrees Fahrenheit for 5 minutes. Place the Oregano Fingers in the fry basket and close it. Let them cook at the same temperature for another 15 minutes or so. Toss the Oregano Fingers well so that they are cooked uniformly.

174. Beef French Toast

Servings: x
Cooking Time: x
Ingredients:
- Bread slices (brown or white)
- 1 egg white for every 2 slices
- 1 tsp sugar for every 2 slices
- ½ lb. sliced beef

Directions:
1. Put two slices together and cut them along the diagonal. In a bowl, whisk the egg whites and add some sugar. Dip the bread triangles into this mixture.
2. Cook the beef now. Pre heat the Kalorik Maxx oven at 180° C for 4 minutes. Place the coated bread triangles in the fry basket and close it. Let them cook at the same temperature for another 20 minutes at least. Halfway through the process, turn the triangles over so that you get a uniform cook. Top with beef and serve.

175. Cayenne Chicken Drumsticks

Servings: 4
Cooking Time: 50 Minutes
Ingredients:
- 8 chicken drumsticks
- 2 tbsp oregano
- 2 tbsp thyme
- 2 oz oats
- ¼ cup milk
- ¼ steamed cauliflower florets
- 1 egg
- 1 tbsp ground cayenne pepper
- Salt and black pepper to taste

Directions:
1. Preheat Kalorik Maxx on Air Fry function to 350 F. Season the drumsticks with salt and pepper; rub them with the milk. Place all the other ingredients except the egg in a food processor. Process until smooth. Dip drumsticks in the egg first and then in the oat mixture. Arrange on the greased AitjrFryer basket and fit in the baking tray. Cook for 20 minutes until golden brown.

176. Calf's Liver Golden Strips

Servings: 4
Cooking Time: 4 To 5 Minutes
Ingredients:
- 1 pound (454 g) sliced calf's liver, cut into about ½-inch-wide strips
- Salt and ground black pepper, to taste
- 2 eggs
- 2 tablespoons milk
- ½ cup whole wheat flour
- 1½ cups panko bread crumbs
- ½ cup plain bread crumbs
- ½ teaspoon salt
- ¼ teaspoon ground black pepper
- Cooking spray

Directions:
1. Sprinkle the liver strips with salt and pepper.
2. Beat together the egg and milk in a bowl. Place wheat flour in a shallow dish. In a second shallow dish, mix panko, plain bread crumbs, ½ teaspoon salt, and ¼ teaspoon pepper.
3. Dip liver strips in flour, egg wash, and then bread crumbs, pressing in coating slightly to make crumbs stick.

4. Spritz the air fryer basket with cooking spray. Place strips in a single layer in the basket.
5. Put the air fryer basket on the baking pan and slide into Rack Position 2, select Air Fry, set the temperature to 400ºF (205ºC) and set the time to 4 minutes.
6. After 2 minutes, remove from the oven. Flip the strips with tongs. Return to the oven and continue cooking.
7. When cooking is complete, the liver strips should be crispy and golden.
8. Serve immediately.

177. Crispy Cracker Crusted Pork Chops

Servings: 3
Cooking Time: 30 Minutes
Ingredients:
- 3 pork chops, boneless
- 2 tbsp milk
- 1 egg, lightly beaten
- 1/2 cup crackers, crushed
- 4 tbsp parmesan cheese, grated
- Pepper
- Salt

Directions:
1. Fit the Kalorik Maxx oven with the rack in position
2. In a shallow bowl, whisk egg and milk.
3. In a separate shallow dish, mix cheese, crackers, pepper, and salt.
4. Dip pork chops in egg then coat with cheese mixture.
5. Place coated pork chops in a baking pan.
6. Set to bake at 350 F for 35 minutes. After 5 minutes place the baking pan in the preheated oven.
7. Serve and enjoy.
- **Nutrition Info:** Calories 360 Fat 25.9 g Carbohydrates 7.2 g Sugar 0.8 g Protein 23.5 g Cholesterol 130 mg

178. Rustic Pork Ribs

Servings: 4
Cooking Time: 15 Minutes
Ingredients:
- 1 rack of pork ribs
- 3 tablespoons dry red wine
- 1 tablespoon soy sauce
- 1/2 teaspoon dried thyme
- 1/2 teaspoon onion powder
- 1/2 teaspoon garlic powder
- 1/2 teaspoon ground black pepper
- 1 teaspoon smoke salt
- 1 tablespoon cornstarch
- 1/2 teaspoon olive oil

Directions:
1. Preparing the Ingredients. Begin by preheating your Kalorik Maxx air fryer oven to 390 degrees F. Place all ingredients in a mixing bowl and let them marinate at least 1 hour.
2. Air Frying. Cook the marinated ribs approximately 25 minutes at 390 degrees F.
3. Serve hot.

179. Mom's Meatballs

Servings: 4
Cooking Time: 20 Minutes
Ingredients:
- 1 lb ground beef
- 2 tbsp olive oil
- 1 red onion, chopped
- 1 garlic clove, minced
- 2 whole eggs, beaten
- Salt and black pepper to taste

Directions:
1. Warm olive oil in a pan over medium heat and sauté onion and garlic for 3 minutes until tender; transfer to a bowl. Add in ground beef and egg and mix well. Season with salt and pepper.
2. Preheat Kalorik Maxx oven to 360 F on AirFry function. Mold the mixture into golf-size ball shapes. Place the balls in the greased frying basket and cook for 12-14 minutes. Serve.

180. Ranch Pork Chops

Servings: 6
Cooking Time: 35 Minutes
Ingredients:
- 6 pork chops, boneless
- 1 tsp dried parsley
- 2 tbsp dry ranch mix
- 1/4 cup olive oil

Directions:
1. Fit the Kalorik Maxx oven with the rack in position
2. Place pork chops in baking dish.
3. Mix together remaining ingredients and pour over pork chops.
4. Set to bake at 425 F for 40 minutes. After 5 minutes place the baking dish in the preheated oven.
5. Serve and enjoy.
- **Nutrition Info:** Calories 330 Fat 28.3 g Carbohydrates 0.4 g Sugar 0 g Protein 18 g Cholesterol 69 mg

181. Crispy Crusted Chicken

Servings: 4
Cooking Time: 30 Minutes
Ingredients:
- 4 chicken breasts, skinless and boneless
- 2 tbsp butter, melted
- 3 cups corn flakes, crushed
- 1 tsp poultry seasoning
- 1 tsp water
- 1 egg, lightly beaten
- Pepper
- Salt

Directions:
1. Fit the Kalorik Maxx oven with the rack in position
2. Season chicken with poultry seasoning, pepper, and salt.
3. In a shallow dish, whisk together egg and water.
4. In a separate shallow dish, mix crushed cornflakes and melted butter.
5. Dip chicken into the egg mixture then coats with crushed cornflakes.
6. Place the coated chicken into the parchment-lined baking pan.
7. Set to bake at 400 F for 35 minutes. After 5 minutes place the baking pan in the preheated oven.
8. Serve and enjoy.
- **Nutrition Info:** Calories 421 Fat 17.7 g Carbohydrates 18.6 g Sugar 1.5 g Protein 45.1 g Cholesterol 186 mg

182. Flavorful Sirloin Steak

Servings: 2
Cooking Time: 14 Minutes
Ingredients:
- 1 lb sirloin steaks
- 1/2 tsp garlic powder
- 1/2 tsp onion powder
- 1/4 tsp smoked paprika
- 1 tsp olive oil
- Pepper
- Salt

Directions:
1. Fit the Kalorik Maxx oven with the rack in position 2.
2. Line the air fryer basket with parchment paper.
3. Brush steak with olive oil and rub with garlic powder, onion powder, paprika, pepper, and salt.
4. Place the steak in the air fryer basket then places an air fryer basket in the baking pan.
5. Place a baking pan on the oven rack. Set to air fry at 400 F for 14 minutes.
6. Serve and enjoy.
- **Nutrition Info:** Calories 447 Fat 16.5 g Carbohydrates 1.2 g Sugar 0.4 g Protein 69 g Cholesterol 203 mg

183. Meatballs(14)

Servings: 4
Cooking Time: 25 Minutes
Ingredients:
- 1 lb ground beef
- 1 tsp fresh rosemary, chopped
- 1 tbsp garlic, chopped
- 1/2 tsp pepper
- 1 tsp garlic powder
- 1 tsp onion powder
- 1/4 cup breadcrumbs
- 2 eggs
- 1 lb ground pork
- 1/2 tsp pepper
- 1 tsp sea salt

Directions:
1. Fit the Kalorik Maxx oven with the rack in position

2. Add all ingredients into the mixing bowl and mix until well combined.
3. Make small balls from the meat mixture and place it into the parchment-lined baking pan.
4. Set to bake at 400 F for 30 minutes. After 5 minutes place the baking pan in the preheated oven.
5. Serve and enjoy.
- **Nutrition Info:** Calories 441 Fat 13.7 g Carbohydrates 7.2 g Sugar 1 g Protein 68.1 g Cholesterol 266 mg

184. Greek Chicken Breast

Servings: 4
Cooking Time: 25 Minutes
Ingredients:
- 4 chicken breasts, skinless & boneless
- 1 tbsp olive oil
- For rub:
- 1 tsp oregano
- 1 tsp thyme
- 1 tsp parsley
- 1 tsp onion powder
- 1 tsp basil
- Pepper
- Salt

Directions:
1. Fit the Kalorik Maxx oven with the rack in position 2.
2. Brush chicken with olive oil.
3. In a small bowl, mix together all rub ingredients and rub all over the chicken breasts.
4. Place chicken into the air fryer basket then places the air fryer basket in the baking pan.
5. Place a baking pan on the oven rack. Set to air fry at 390 F for 25 minutes.
6. Serve and enjoy.
- **Nutrition Info:** Calories 312 Fat 14.4 g Carbohydrates 0.9 g Sugar 0.2 g Protein 42.4 g Cholesterol 130 mg

185. Chicken Madeira

Servings: x
Cooking Time: x
Ingredients:
- 2 cups Madeira wine
- 2 cups beef broth
- ½ cup shredded Mozzarella cheese
- 4 boneless, skinless chicken breasts
- 1 Tbsp salt
- Salt and freshly ground black pepper, to taste
- 6 cups water
- ½ lb. asparagus, trimmed
- 2 Tbsp extra-virgin olive oil
- 2 Tbsp chopped fresh parsley

Directions:
1. Lay the chicken breasts on a cutting board, and cover each with a piece of plastic wrap. Use a mallet or a small, heavy frying pan to pound them to ¼ inch thick. Discard the plastic wrap and season with salt and pepper on both sides of the chicken.
2. Fill Kalorik Maxx oven with the water, bring to a boil, and add the salt.
3. Add the asparagus and boil, uncovered, until crisp, tender, and bright green, 2 to 3 minutes. Remove immediately and set aside. Pour out the water.
4. In Kalorik Maxx oven over medium heat, heat the olive oil. Cook the chicken for 4 to 5 minutes on each side. Remove and set aside.
5. Add the Madeira wine and beef broth. Bring to a boil, reduce to a simmer, and cook for 10 to 12 minutes.
6. Return the chicken to the pot, turning it to coat in the sauce.
7. Lay the asparagus and cheese on top of the chicken. Then transfer Kalorik Maxx oven to the oven broiler and broil for 3 to 4 minutes. Garnish with the parsley, if using, and serve.

186. Air Fry Chicken Drumsticks

Servings: 6
Cooking Time: 25 Minutes
Ingredients:
- 6 chicken drumsticks
- 1/2 tsp garlic powder
- 2 tbsp olive oil
- 1/2 tsp ground cumin
- 3/4 tsp paprika
- Pepper
- Salt

Directions:

1. Fit the Kalorik Maxx oven with the rack in position 2.
2. Add chicken drumsticks and olive oil in a large bowl and toss well.
3. Sprinkle garlic powder, paprika, cumin, pepper, and salt over chicken drumsticks and toss until well coated.
4. Place chicken drumsticks in the air fryer basket then place an air fryer basket in the baking pan.
5. Place a baking pan on the oven rack. Set to air fry at 400 F for 25 minutes.
6. Serve and enjoy.
- **Nutrition Info:** Calories 120 Fat 7.4 g Carbohydrates 0.4 g Sugar 0.1 g Protein 12.8 g Cholesterol 40 mg

187. Lime-chili Chicken Wings

Servings: 2
Cooking Time: 25 Minutes
Ingredients:
- 9 chicken wings
- 2 tbsp hot chili sauce
- ½ tbsp lime juice
- ½ tbsp honey
- ½ tbsp kosher salt
- ½ tbsp black pepper

Directions:
1. Preheat Kalorik Maxx on Air Fry function to 350 F. Mix the lime juice, honey, and chili sauce. Toss the mixture over the chicken wings. Put the chicken wings in the basket and fit in the baking tray; cook for 25 minutes. Shake every 5 minutes. Serve.

188. Ham Flat Cakes

Servings: x
Cooking Time: x
Ingredients:
- 2 tbsp. garam masala
- 1 lb. thinly sliced ham
- 3 tsp ginger finely chopped
- 1-2 tbsp. fresh coriander leaves
- 2 or 3 green chilies finely chopped
- 1 ½ tbsp. lemon juice
- Salt and pepper to taste

Directions:

1. Mix the ingredients in a clean bowl and add water to it. Make sure that the paste is not too watery but is enough to apply on the sides of the ham slices.
2. Pre heat the Kalorik Maxx oven at 160 degrees Fahrenheit for 5 minutes. Place the French Cuisine Galettes in the fry basket and let them cook for another 25 minutes at the same temperature. Keep rolling them over to get a uniform cook. Serve either with mint sauce or ketchup.

189. Corn Flour Lamb Fries With Red Chili

Servings: x
Cooking Time: x
Ingredients:
- 2 tsp. salt
- 1 tsp. pepper powder
- 1 lb. boneless lamb cut into Oregano Fingers
- 2 cup dry breadcrumbs
- 2 tsp. oregano
- 2 tsp. red chili flakes
- 1 ½ tbsp. ginger-garlic paste
- 4 tbsp. lemon juice
- 1 tsp. red chili powder
- 6 tbsp. corn flour
- 4 eggs

Directions:
1. Mix all the ingredients for the marinade and put the lamb Oregano Fingers inside and let it rest overnight.
2. Mix the breadcrumbs, oregano and red chili flakes well and place the
3. marinated Oregano Fingers on this mixture. Cover it with plastic wrap and leave it till right before you serve to cook.
4. Pre heat the Kalorik Maxx oven at 160 degrees Fahrenheit for 5 minutes. Place the Oregano Fingers in the fry basket and close it. Let them cook at the same temperature for another 15 minutes or so. Toss the Oregano Fingers well so that they are cooked uniformly.

190. Smoky Paprika Pork And Vegetable Kabobs

Servings: 4
Cooking Time: 15 Minutes

Ingredients:
- 1 pound (454 g) pork tenderloin, cubed
- 1 teaspoon smoked paprika
- Salt and ground black pepper, to taste
- 1 green bell pepper, cut into chunks
- 1 zucchini, cut into chunks
- 1 red onion, sliced
- 1 tablespoon oregano
- Cooking spray
- Special Equipment:
- Small bamboo skewers, soaked in water for 20 minutes to keep them from burning while cooking

Directions:
1. Spritz the air fryer basket with cooking spray.
2. Add the pork to a bowl and season with the smoked paprika, salt and black pepper. Thread the seasoned pork cubes and vegetables alternately onto the soaked skewers. Arrange the skewers in the pan.
3. Put the air fryer basket on the baking pan and slide into Rack Position 2, select Air Fry, set temperature to 350ºF (180ºC) and set time to 15 minutes.
4. After 7 minutes, remove from the oven. Flip the pork skewers. Return to the oven and continue cooking.
5. When cooking is complete, the pork should be browned and vegetables are tender.
6. Transfer the skewers to the serving dishes and sprinkle with oregano. Serve hot.

191. Turkey Grandma's Easy To Cook Wontons

Servings: x
Cooking Time: x
Ingredients:
- 1 ½ cup all-purpose flour
- ½ tsp. salt
- 5 tbsp. water
- 2 cups minced turkey
- 2 tbsp. oil
- 2 tsp. ginger-garlic paste
- 2 tsp. soya sauce
- 2 tsp. vinegar

Directions:
1. Squeeze the dough and cover it with plastic wrap and set aside. Next, cook the ingredients for the filling and try to ensure that the turkey is covered well with the sauce. Roll the dough and place the filling in the center. Now, wrap the dough to cover the filling and pinch the edges together. Pre heat the Kalorik Maxx oven at 200° F for 5 minutes.
2. Place the wontons in the fry basket and close it. Let them cook at the same temperature for another 20 minutes. Recommended sides are chili sauce or ketchup.

192. Grandma's Ground Beef Balls

Servings: 4
Cooking Time: 15 Minutes
Ingredients:
- 1 pound ground beef
- 1 tbsp olive oil
- 1 large red onion, chopped
- 1 tsp garlic, minced
- 2 whole eggs, beaten
- Salt and black pepper to taste

Directions:
1. Place a skillet over medium heat and warm the oil. Add in onion and garlic and sauté for 3 minutes until tender. Remove to a bowl to cool. Add in the ground beef and egg and mix well.
2. Season with salt and pepper. Roll the mixture into golf-sized balls and place them in the greased frying basket. Fit in the baking tray and cook for 15 minutes on Air Fry function at 350 F. Serve.

193. Caraway Crusted Beef Steaks

Servings: 4
Cooking Time: 10 Minutes
Ingredients:
- 4 beef steaks
- 2 teaspoons caraway seeds
- 2 teaspoons garlic powder
- Sea salt and cayenne pepper, to taste
- 1 tablespoon melted butter
- $1/3$ cup almond flour
- 2 eggs, beaten

Directions:
1. Add the beef steaks to a large bowl and toss with the caraway seeds, garlic powder, salt and pepper until well coated.
2. Stir together the melted butter and almond flour in a bowl. Whisk the eggs in a different bowl.
3. Dredge the seasoned steaks in the eggs, then dip in the almond and butter mixture.
4. Arrange the coated steaks in the basket.
5. Put the air fryer basket on the baking pan and slide into Rack Position 2, select Air Fry, set temperature to 355ºF (179ºC) and set time to 10 minutes.
6. Flip the steaks once halfway through to ensure even cooking.
7. When cooking is complete, the internal temperature of the beef steaks should reach at least 145ºF (63ºC) on a meat thermometer.
8. Transfer the steaks to plates. Let cool for 5 minutes and serve hot.

194. Chicken Skewers With Corn Salad

Servings: 4
Cooking Time: 10 Minutes
Ingredients:
- 1 pound (454 g) boneless, skinless chicken breast, cut into 1½-inch chunks
- 1 green bell pepper, deseeded and cut into 1-inch pieces
- 1 red bell pepper, deseeded and cut into 1-inch pieces
- 1 large onion, cut into large chunks
- 2 tablespoons fajita seasoning
- 3 tablespoons vegetable oil, divided
- 2 teaspoons kosher salt, divided
- 2 cups corn, drained
- ¼ teaspoon granulated garlic
- 1 teaspoon freshly squeezed lime juice
- 1 tablespoon mayonnaise
- 3 tablespoons grated Parmesan cheese
- Special Equipment:
- 12 wooden skewers, soaked in water for at least 30 minutes

Directions:
1. Place the chicken, bell peppers, and onion in a large bowl. Add the fajita seasoning, 2 tablespoons of vegetable oil, and 1½ teaspoons of kosher salt. Toss to coat evenly.
2. Alternate the chicken and vegetables on the skewers, making about 12 skewers.
3. Place the corn in a medium bowl and add the remaining vegetable oil. Add the remaining kosher salt and the garlic, and toss to coat. Place the corn in an even layer in the baking pan and place the skewers on top.
4. Slide the baking pan into Rack Position 2, select Roast, set temperature to 375ºF (190ºC), and set time to 10 minutes.
5. After about 5 minutes, remove from the oven and turn the skewers. Return to the oven and continue cooking.
6. When cooking is complete, remove from the oven. Place the skewers on a platter. Put the corn back to the bowl and combine with the lime juice, mayonnaise, and Parmesan cheese. Stir to mix well. Serve the skewers with the corn.

195. Parmesan Chicken Cutlets

Servings: 4
Cooking Time: 30 Minutes
Ingredients:
- ¼ cup Parmesan cheese, grated
- 4 chicken cutlets
- ⅛ tbsp paprika
- 2 tbsp panko breadcrumbs
- ½ tbsp garlic powder
- 2 large eggs, beaten

Directions:
1. In a bowl, mix Parmesan cheese, breadcrumbs, garlic powder, and paprika. Add eggs to another bowl. Dip the chicken in eggs, dredge them in cheese mixture and place them in the basket and fit in the baking tray. Cook for 20-25 minutes on Air Fry function at 400 F.

FISH & SEAFOOD RECIPES

196. Breaded Fish Fillets

Servings: 4
Cooking Time: 7 Minutes
Ingredients:
- 1 pound (454 g) fish fillets
- 1 tablespoon coarse brown mustard
- 1 teaspoon Worcestershire sauce
- ½ teaspoon hot sauce
- Salt, to taste
- Cooking spray
- Crumb Coating:
- ¾ cup panko bread crumbs
- ¼ cup stone-ground cornmeal
- ¼ teaspoon salt

Directions:
1. On your cutting board, cut the fish fillets crosswise into slices, about 1 inch wide.
2. In a small bowl, stir together the mustard, Worcestershire sauce, and hot sauce to make a paste and rub this paste on all sides of the fillets. Season with salt to taste.
3. In a shallow bowl, thoroughly combine all the ingredients for the crumb coating and spread them on a sheet of wax paper.
4. Roll the fish fillets in the crumb mixture until thickly coated. Spritz all sides of the fish with cooking spray, then arrange them in the air fryer basket in a single layer.
5. Put the air fryer basket on the baking pan and slide into Rack Position 2, select Air Fry, set temperature to 400ºF (205ºC), and set time to 7 minutes.
6. When cooking is complete, the fish should flake apart with a fork. Remove from the oven and serve warm.

197. Tomato Garlic Shrimp

Servings: 4
Cooking Time: 25 Minutes
Ingredients:
- 1 lb shrimp, peeled
- 1 tbsp garlic, sliced
- 2 cups cherry tomatoes
- 1 tbsp olive oil
- Pepper
- Salt

Directions:
1. Fit the Kalorik Maxx oven with the rack in position
2. Add shrimp, oil, garlic, tomatoes, pepper, and salt into the large bowl and toss well.
3. Transfer shrimp mixture into the baking dish.
4. Set to bake at 400 F for 30 minutes. After 5 minutes place the baking dish in the preheated oven.
5. Serve and enjoy.
- **Nutrition Info:** Calories 184 Fat 5.6 g Carbohydrates 5.9 g Sugar 2.4 g Protein 26.8 gCholesterol 239 mg

198. Tuna Sandwich

Servings: x
Cooking Time: x
Ingredients:
- 2 slices of white bread
- 1 tbsp. softened butter
- 1 tin tuna
- 1 small capsicum
- For Barbeque Sauce:
- ¼ tbsp. Worcestershire sauce
- ½ tsp. olive oil
- ¼ tsp. mustard powder
- ½ flake garlic crushed
- ¼ cup chopped onion
- ½ tbsp. sugar
- 1 tbsp. tomato ketchup
- ½ cup water.
- ¼ tbsp. red chili sauce
- A pinch of salt and black pepper to taste

Directions:
1. Take the slices of bread and remove the edges. Now cut the slices horizontally. Cook the ingredients for the sauce and wait till it thickens. Now, add the lamb to the sauce and stir till it obtains the flavors. Roast the capsicum and peel the skin off. Cut the capsicum into slices. Mix the ingredients together and apply it to the bread slices.
2. Pre-heat the Kalorik Maxx oven for 5 minutes at 300 Fahrenheit. Open the basket of the Fryer and place the prepared Classic

Sandwiches in it such that no two Classic Sandwiches are touching each other. Now keep the fryer at 250 degrees for around 15 minutes. Turn the Classic Sandwiches in between the cooking process to cook both slices. Serve the Classic Sandwiches with tomato ketchup or mint sauce.

199. Old Bay Crab Cakes

Servings: 4
Cooking Time: 20 Minutes
Ingredients:
- 2 slices dried bread, crusts removed
- Small amount of milk
- 1 tablespoon mayonnaise
- 1 tablespoon Worcestershire sauce
- 1 tablespoon baking powder
- 1 tablespoon parsley flakes
- 1 teaspoon Old Bay® Seasoning
- 1/4 teaspoon salt
- 1 egg
- 1 pound lump crabmeat

Directions:
1. Preparing the Ingredients. Crush your bread over a large bowl until it is broken down into small pieces. Add milk and stir until bread crumbs are moistened. Mix in mayo and Worcestershire sauce. Add remaining ingredients and mix well. Shape into 4 patties.
2. Air Frying. Cook at 360 degrees for 20 minutes, flip half way through.
- **Nutrition Info:** CALORIES: 165; CARBS:5.8; FAT: 4.5G; PROTEIN:24G; FIBER:0G

200. Rosemary Buttered Prawns

Servings: 2
Cooking Time: 15 Minutes + Marinating Time
Ingredients:
- 8 large prawns
- 1 rosemary sprig, chopped
- ½ tbsp melted butter
- Salt and black pepper to taste

Directions:
1. Combine butter, rosemary, salt, and pepper in a bowl. Add in the prawns and mix to coat. Cover the bowl and refrigerate for 1 hour.
2. Preheat Kalorik Maxx on Air Fry function to 350 F Remove the prawns from the fridge and place them in the basket. Fit in the baking tray and cook for 10 minutes, flipping once. Serve.

201. Crispy Paprika Fish Fillets(1)

Servings: 4
Cooking Time: 15 Minutes
Ingredients:
- 1/2 cup seasoned breadcrumbs
- 1 tablespoon balsamic vinegar
- 1/2 teaspoon seasoned salt
- 1 teaspoon paprika
- 1/2 teaspoon ground black pepper
- 1 teaspoon celery seed
- 2 fish fillets, halved
- 1 egg, beaten

Directions:
1. Preparing the Ingredients. Add the breadcrumbs, vinegar, salt, paprika, ground black pepper, and celery seeds to your food processor. Process for about 30 seconds.
2. Coat the fish fillets with the beaten egg; then, coat them with the breadcrumbs mixture.
3. Air Frying. Cook at 350 degrees F for about 15 minutes.

202. Prawn French Cuisine Galette

Servings:x
Cooking Time:x
Ingredients:
- 2 tbsp. garam masala
- 1 lb. minced prawn
- 3 tsp ginger finely chopped
- 1-2 tbsp. fresh coriander leaves
- 2 or 3 green chilies finely chopped
- 1 ½ tbsp. lemon juice
- Salt and pepper to taste

Directions:
1. Mix the ingredients in a clean bowl.
2. Mold this mixture into round and flat French Cuisine Galettes.
3. Wet the French Cuisine Galettes slightly with water.
4. Pre heat the Kalorik Maxx oven at 160 degrees Fahrenheit for 5 minutes. Place the

French Cuisine Galettes in the fry basket and let them cook for another 25 minutes at the same temperature. Keep rolling them over to get a uniform cook. Serve either with mint sauce or ketchup.

203. Crispy Salmon With Lemon-butter Sauce

Servings: x
Cooking Time: x
Ingredients:
- 4 (4-6-oz) salmon fillets, patted dry
- Salt and pepper, to taste
- 2 Tbsp olive oil
- 1 large garlic clove, minced
- 1/3 cup dry white wine
- 2 Tbsp fresh lemon juice
- 1 lemon zested
- 3 Tbsp unsalted butter, diced
- 2 Tbsp chopped fresh dill

Directions:
1. Place Kalorik Maxx oven over medium heat.
2. Sprinkle salt and pepper on salmon fillets and add 1 Tbsp oil to the pan.
3. Add salmon flesh side down and cook 3-4 minutes. Flip the salmon and cook an additional 3 minutes on skin side. Transfer to a plate.
4. Wipe out Kalorik Maxx oven and add remaining Tbsp olive oil over medium heat.
5. Add garlic and saute for 1 minute.
6. Pour in white wine and lemon juice. Stir for one minute.
7. Add lemon zest and continue stirring until slightly reduced.
8. Reduce heat to low and add cubed butter, stirring after each addition.
9. Sprinkle in fresh dill and stir all together.
10. Season with salt and pepper and pour sauce over salmon fillets.

204. Basil White Fish

Servings: 4
Cooking Time: 20 Minutes
Ingredients:
- 2 tbsp fresh basil, chopped
- 2 garlic cloves, minced
- 1 tbsp Parmesan cheese, grated
- Salt and black pepper to taste
- 2 tbsp pine nuts
- 4 white fish fillets
- 2 tbsp olive oil

Directions:
1. Preheat Kalorik Maxx on AirFry function to 350 F. Season the fillets with salt and pepper and place in the basket. Drizzle with some olive oil and press Start. Cook for 12-14 minutes. In a bowl, mix basil, remaining olive oil, pine nuts, garlic, and Parmesan cheese and spread on the fish. Serve.

205. Baked Tilapia With Garlic Aioli

Servings: 4
Cooking Time: 15 Minutes
Ingredients:
- Tilapia:
- 4 tilapia fillets
- 1 tablespoon extra-virgin olive oil
- 1 teaspoon garlic powder
- 1 teaspoon paprika
- 1 teaspoon dried basil
- A pinch of lemon-pepper seasoning
- Garlic Aioli:
- 2 garlic cloves, minced
- 1 tablespoon mayonnaise
- Juice of ½ lemon
- 1 teaspoon extra-virgin olive oil
- Salt and pepper, to taste

Directions:
1. On a clean work surface, brush both sides of each fillet with the olive oil. Sprinkle with the garlic powder, paprika, basil, and lemon-pepper seasoning. Place the fillets in the baking pan.
2. Slide the baking pan into Rack Position 1, select Convection Bake, set temperature to 400ºF (205ºC), and set time to 15 minutes.
3. Flip the fillets halfway through.
4. Meanwhile, make the garlic aioli: Whisk together the garlic, mayo, lemon juice, olive oil, salt, and pepper in a small bowl until smooth.
5. When cooking is complete, the fish should flake apart with a fork and no longer translucent in the center. Remove the fish

from the oven and serve with the garlic aioli on the side.

206. Fish Club Classic Sandwich

Servings: x
Cooking Time: x
Ingredients:
- 2 slices of white bread
- 1 tbsp. softened butter
- 1 tin tuna
- 1 small capsicum
- For Barbeque Sauce:
- ¼ tbsp. Worcestershire sauce
- ½ tsp. olive oil
- ½ flake garlic crushed
- ¼ cup chopped onion
- ¼ tsp. mustard powder
- ½ tbsp. sugar
- ¼ tbsp. red chili sauce
- 1 tbsp. tomato ketchup
- ½ cup water.
- A pinch of salt and black pepper to taste

Directions:
1. Take the slices of bread and remove the edges. Now cut the slices horizontally. Cook the ingredients for the sauce and wait till it thickens. Now, add the fish to the sauce and stir till it obtains the flavors. Roast the capsicum and peel the skin off. Cut the capsicum into slices.
2. Mix the ingredients together and apply it to the bread slices. Pre-heat the Kalorik Maxx oven for 5 minutes at 300 Fahrenheit.
3. Open the basket of the Fryer and place the prepared Classic Sandwiches in it such that no two Classic Sandwiches are touching each other. Now keep the fryer at 250 degrees for around 15 minutes. Turn the Classic Sandwiches in between the cooking process to cook both slices. Serve the Classic Sandwiches with tomato ketchup or mint sauce.

207. Lemon Butter Shrimp

Servings: 4
Cooking Time: 12 Minutes
Ingredients:
- 1 1/4 lbs shrimp, peeled & deveined
- 2 tbsp fresh parsley, chopped
- 2 tbsp fresh lemon juice
- 1 tbsp garlic, minced
- 1/4 cup butter
- Pepper
- Salt

Directions:
1. Fit the Kalorik Maxx oven with the rack in position
2. Add shrimp into the baking dish.
3. Melt butter in a pan over low heat. Add garlic and sauté for 30 seconds. Stir in lemon juice.
4. Pour melted butter mixture over shrimp. Season with pepper and salt.
5. Set to bake at 350 F for 17 minutes. After 5 minutes place the baking dish in the preheated oven.
6. Garnish with parsley and serve.
- **Nutrition Info:** Calories 276 Fat 14 g Carbohydrates 3.2 g Sugar 0.2 g Protein 32.7 g Cholesterol 329 mg

208. Cheese Carp Fries

Servings: x
Cooking Time: x
Ingredients:
- 1 lb. carp Oregano Fingers
- ingredients for the marinade:
- 1 tbsp. olive oil
- 1 tsp. mixed herbs
- ½ tsp. red chili flakes
- A pinch of salt to taste
- 1 tbsp. lemon juice
- For the garnish:
- 1 cup melted cheddar cheese

Directions:
1. Take all the ingredients mentioned under the heading "For the marinade" and mix them well. Cook the carp Oregano Fingers and soak them in the marinade.
2. Pre heat the Kalorik Maxx oven for around 5 minutes at 300 Fahrenheit. Take out the basket of the fryer and place the carp in them. Close the basket. Now keep the fryer at 220 Fahrenheit for 20 or 25 minutes.
3. In between the process, toss the fries twice or thrice so that they get cooked properly.

Towards the end of the cooking process (the last 2 minutes or so), sprinkle the melted cheddar cheese over the fries and serve hot.

209. Basil Salmon With Tomatoes

Servings: 4
Cooking Time: 15 Minutes
Ingredients:
- 4 (6-ounce / 170-g) salmon fillets, patted dry
- 1 teaspoon kosher salt, divided
- 2 pints cherry or grape tomatoes, halved if large, divided
- 3 tablespoons extra-virgin olive oil, divided
- 2 garlic cloves, minced
- 1 small red bell pepper, deseeded and chopped
- 2 tablespoons chopped fresh basil, divided

Directions:
1. Season both sides of the salmon with ½ teaspoon of kosher salt.
2. Put about half of the tomatoes in a large bowl, along with the remaining ½ teaspoon of kosher salt, 2 tablespoons of olive oil, garlic, bell pepper, and 1 tablespoon of basil. Toss to coat and then transfer to the baking pan.
3. Arrange the salmon fillets in the pan, skin-side down. Brush them with the remaining 1 tablespoon of olive oil.
4. Slide the baking pan into Rack Position 2, select Roast, set temperature to 375ºF (190ºC), and set time to 15 minutes.
5. After 7 minutes, remove the pan and fold in the remaining tomatoes. Return the pan to the oven and continue cooking.
6. When cooked, remove from the oven. Serve sprinkled with the remaining 1 tablespoon of basil.

210. Tuna Lettuce Wraps

Servings: 4
Cooking Time: 4 To 7 Minutes
Ingredients:
- 1 pound (454 g) fresh tuna steak, cut into 1-inch cubes
- 2 garlic cloves, minced
- 1 tablespoon grated fresh ginger
- ½ teaspoon toasted sesame oil
- 4 low-sodium whole-wheat tortillas
- 2 cups shredded romaine lettuce
- 1 red bell pepper, thinly sliced
- ¼ cup low-fat mayonnaise

Directions:
1. Combine the tuna cubes, garlic, ginger, and sesame oil in a medium bowl and toss until well coated. Allow to sit for 10 minutes.
2. When ready, place the tuna cubes in the air fryer basket.
3. Put the air fryer basket on the baking pan and slide into Rack Position 2, select Air Fry, set temperature to 390ºF (199ºC), and set time to 6 minutes.
4. When cooking is complete, the tuna cubes should be cooked through and golden brown. Remove the tuna cubes from the oven to a plate.
5. Make the wraps: Place the tortillas on a flat work surface and top each tortilla evenly with the cooked tuna, lettuce, bell pepper, and finish with the mayonnaise. Roll them up and serve immediately.

211. Baked Pesto Salmon

Servings: 4
Cooking Time: 15 Minutes
Ingredients:
- 4 salmon fillets
- 1/3 cup parmesan cheese, grated
- 1/3 cup breadcrumbs
- 6 tbsp pesto

Directions:
1. Fit the Kalorik Maxx oven with the rack in position
2. Place fish fillets into the baking dish.
3. Pour pesto over fish fillets.
4. Mix together breadcrumbs and parmesan cheese and sprinkle over fish.
5. Set to bake at 325 F for 20 minutes. After 5 minutes place the baking dish in the preheated oven.
6. Serve and enjoy.
- **Nutrition Info:** Calories 396 Fat 22.8 g Carbohydrates 8.3 g Sugar 2.1 g Protein 40.4 g Cholesterol 89 mg

212. Tasty Parmesan Shrimp

Servings: 4
Cooking Time: 10 Minutes
Ingredients:
- 1 lb shrimp, peeled and deveined
- 1/4 cup parmesan cheese, grated
- 4 garlic cloves, minced
- 1 tbsp olive oil
- 1/4 tsp oregano
- 1/2 tsp pepper
- 1/2 tsp onion powder
- 1/2 tsp basil

Directions:
1. Fit the Kalorik Maxx oven with the rack in position 2.
2. Add all ingredients into the large bowl and toss well.
3. Add shrimp to the air fryer basket then place an air fryer basket in the baking pan.
4. Place a baking pan on the oven rack. Set to air fry at 350 F for 10 minutes.
5. Serve and enjoy.
- **Nutrition Info:** Calories 189 Fat 6.7 g Carbohydrates 3.4 g Sugar 0.1 g Protein 27.9 g Cholesterol 243 mg

213. Crispy Paprika Fish Fillets(2)

Servings: 4
Cooking Time: 15 Minutes
Ingredients:
- 1/2 cup seasoned breadcrumbs
- 1 tablespoon balsamic vinegar
- 1/2 teaspoon seasoned salt
- 1 teaspoon paprika
- 1/2 teaspoon ground black pepper
- 1 teaspoon celery seed
- 2 fish fillets, halved
- 1 egg, beaten

Directions:
1. Preparing the Ingredients. Add the breadcrumbs, vinegar, salt, paprika, ground black pepper, and celery seeds to your food processor. Process for about 30 seconds.
2. Coat the fish fillets with the beaten egg; then, coat them with the breadcrumbs mixture.
3. Air Frying. Cook at 350 degrees F for about 15 minutes.

214. Fish Spicy Lemon Kebab

Servings: x
Cooking Time: x
Ingredients:
- 1 lb. boneless fish roughly chopped
- 3 onions chopped
- 5 green chilies-roughly chopped
- 1 ½ tbsp. ginger paste
- 1 ½ tsp garlic paste
- 1 ½ tsp salt
- 3 tsp lemon juice
- 2 tsp garam masala
- 4 tbsp. chopped coriander
- 3 tbsp. cream
- 2 tbsp. coriander powder
- 4 tbsp. fresh mint chopped
- 3 tbsp. chopped capsicum
- 3 eggs
- 2 ½ tbsp. white sesame seeds

Directions:
1. Take all the ingredients mentioned under the first heading and mix them in a bowl. Grind them thoroughly to make a smooth paste. Take the eggs in a different bowl and beat them. Add a pinch of salt and leave them aside. Take a flat plate and in it mix the sesame seeds and breadcrumbs. Mold the fish mixture into small balls and flatten them into round and flat kebabs. Dip these kebabs in the egg and salt mixture and then in the mixture of breadcrumbs and sesame seeds. Leave these kebabs in the fridge for an hour or so to set.
2. Pre heat the Kalorik Maxx oven at 160 degrees Fahrenheit for around 5 minutes. Place the kebabs in the basket and let them cook for another 25 minutes at the same temperature. Turn the kebabs over in between the cooking process to get a uniform cook. Serve the kebabs with mint sauce.

215. Shrimp And Cherry Tomato Kebabs

Servings: 4
Cooking Time: 5 Minutes

Ingredients:
- 1½ pounds (680 g) jumbo shrimp, cleaned, shelled and deveined
- 1 pound (454 g) cherry tomatoes
- 2 tablespoons butter, melted
- 1 tablespoons Sriracha sauce
- Sea salt and ground black pepper, to taste
- 1 teaspoon dried parsley flakes
- ½ teaspoon dried basil
- ½ teaspoon dried oregano
- ½ teaspoon mustard seeds
- ½ teaspoon marjoram
- Special Equipment:
- 4 to 6 wooden skewers, soaked in water for 30 minutes

Directions:
1. Put all the ingredients in a large bowl and toss to coat well.
2. Make the kebabs: Thread, alternating jumbo shrimp and cherry tomatoes, onto the wooden skewers. Place the kebabs in the air fryer basket.
3. Put the air fryer basket on the baking pan and slide into Rack Position 2, select Air Fry, set temperature to 400ºF (205ºC), and set time to 5 minutes.
4. When cooking is complete, the shrimp should be pink and the cherry tomatoes should be softened. Remove from the oven. Let the shrimp and cherry tomato kebabs cool for 5 minutes and serve hot.

216. Easy Scallops

Servings: 2
Cooking Time: 4 Minutes
Ingredients:
- 12 medium sea scallops, rinsed and patted dry
- 1 teaspoon fine sea salt
- ¾ teaspoon ground black pepper, plus more for garnish
- Fresh thyme leaves, for garnish (optional)
- Avocado oil spray

Directions:
1. Coat the air fryer basket with avocado oil spray.
2. Place the scallops in a medium bowl and spritz with avocado oil spray. Sprinkle the salt and pepper to season.
3. Transfer the seasoned scallops to the basket, spacing them apart.
4. Put the air fryer basket on the baking pan and slide into Rack Position 2, select Air Fry, set temperature to 390ºF (199ºC), and set time to 4 minutes.
5. Flip the scallops halfway through the cooking time.
6. When cooking is complete, the scallops should reach an internal temperature of just 145ºF (63ºC) on a meat thermometer. Sprinkle the pepper and thyme leaves on top for garnish, if desired. Serve immediately.

217. Herb Baked Catfish Fillets

Servings: 4
Cooking Time: 20 Minutes
Ingredients:
- 4 catfish fillets
- 1/2 tsp garlic powder
- 2 tbsp butter, melted
- 1 lemon juice
- 1/2 tsp pepper
- 1/2 tsp dried basil
- 1/2 tsp dried thyme
- 3/4 tsp paprika
- 1/2 tsp dried oregano
- 1 tsp salt

Directions:
1. Fit the Kalorik Maxx oven with the rack in position
2. Place fish fillets into the baking pan.
3. Mix together garlic powder, pepper, basil, oregano, thyme, paprika, and salt and sprinkle over fish fillets.
4. Pour lemon juice and melted butter over fish fillets.
5. Set to bake at 350 F for 25 minutes. After 5 minutes place the baking pan in the preheated oven.
6. Serve and enjoy.
- **Nutrition Info:** Calories 274 Fat 18.1 g Carbohydrates 1.1 g Sugar 0.4 g Protein 25.2 g Cholesterol 90 mg

218. Cajun Catfish Cakes With Cheese

Servings: 4
Cooking Time: 15 Minutes
Ingredients:
- 2 catfish fillets
- 3 ounces (85 g) butter
- 1 cup shredded Parmesan cheese
- 1 cup shredded Swiss cheese
- ½ cup buttermilk
- 1 teaspoon baking powder
- 1 teaspoon baking soda
- 1 teaspoon Cajun seasoning

Directions:
1. Bring a pot of salted water to a boil. Add the catfish fillets to the boiling water and let them boil for 5 minutes until they become opaque.
2. Remove the fillets from the pot to a mixing bowl and flake them into small pieces with a fork.
3. Add the remaining ingredients to the bowl of fish and stir until well incorporated.
4. Divide the fish mixture into 12 equal portions and shape each portion into a patty. Place the patties in the air fryer basket.
5. Put the air fryer basket on the baking pan and slide into Rack Position 2, select Air Fry, set temperature to 380ºF (193ºC), and set time to 15 minutes.
6. Flip the patties halfway through the cooking time.
7. When cooking is complete, the patties should be golden brown and cooked through. Remove from the oven. Let the patties sit for 5 minutes and serve.

219. Spinach & Tuna Balls With Ricotta

Servings: 4
Cooking Time: 20 Minutes
Ingredients:
- 14 oz store-bought crescent dough
- ½ cup spinach, steamed
- 1 cup ricotta cheese, crumbled
- ¼ tsp garlic powder
- 1 tsp fresh oregano, chopped
- ½ cup canned tuna, drained

Directions:
1. Preheat Kalorik Maxx on AirFry function to 350 F. Roll the dough onto a lightly floured flat surface. Combine the ricotta cheese, spinach, tuna, oregano, salt, and garlic powder together in a bowl.
2. Cut the dough into 4 equal pieces. Divide the mixture between the dough pieces. Make sure to place the filling in the center. Fold the dough and secure with a fork. Place onto a lined baking dish and press Start. Cook for 12 minutes until lightly browned. Serve.

220. Panko Crab Sticks With Mayo Sauce

Servings: 4
Cooking Time: 12 Minutes
Ingredients:
- Crab Sticks:
- 2 eggs
- 1 cup flour
- ⅓ cup panko bread crumbs
- 1 tablespoon old bay seasoning
- 1 pound (454 g) crab sticks
- Cooking spray
- Mayo Sauce:
- ½ cup mayonnaise
- 1 lime, juiced
- 2 garlic cloves, minced

Directions:
1. In a bowl, beat the eggs. In a shallow bowl, place the flour. In another shallow bowl, thoroughly combine the panko bread crumbs and old bay seasoning.
2. Dredge the crab sticks in the flour, shaking off any excess, then in the beaten eggs, finally press them in the bread crumb mixture to coat well.
3. Arrange the crab sticks in the air fryer basket and spray with cooking spray.
4. Put the air fryer basket on the baking pan and slide into Rack Position 2, select Air Fry, set temperature to 390ºF (199ºC), and set time to 12 minutes.
5. Flip the crab sticks halfway through the cooking time.

6. Meanwhile, make the sauce by whisking together the mayo, lime juice, and garlic in a small bowl.
7. When cooking is complete, remove from the oven. Serve the crab sticks with the mayo sauce on the side.

221. Garlic Butter Shrimp Scampi

Servings: 4
Cooking Time: 8 Minutes
Ingredients:
- Sauce:
- ¼ cup unsalted butter
- 2 tablespoons fish stock or chicken broth
- 2 cloves garlic, minced
- 2 tablespoons chopped fresh basil leaves
- 1 tablespoon lemon juice
- 1 tablespoon chopped fresh parsley, plus more for garnish
- 1 teaspoon red pepper flakes
- Shrimp:
- 1 pound (454 g) large shrimp, peeled and deveined, tails removed
- Fresh basil sprigs, for garnish

Directions:
1. Put all the ingredients for the sauce in the baking pan and stir to incorporate.
2. Put the air fryer basket on the baking pan and slide into Rack Position 2, select Air Fry, set temperature to 350ºF (180ºC), and set time to 8 minutes.
3. After 3 minutes, remove from the oven and add the shrimp to the baking pan, flipping to coat in the sauce. Return to the oven and continue cooking for 5 minutes until the shrimp are pink and opaque. Stir the shrimp twice during cooking.
4. When cooking is complete, remove from the oven. Serve garnished with the parsley and basil sprigs.

222. Tasty Tuna Loaf

Servings: 6
Cooking Time: 40 Minutes
Ingredients:
- Nonstick cooking spray
- 12 oz. can chunk white tuna in water, drain & flake
- ¾ cup bread crumbs
- 1 onion, chopped fine
- 2 eggs, beaten
- ¼ cup milk
- ½ tsp fresh lemon juice
- ½ tsp dill
- 1 tbsp. fresh parsley, chopped
- ½ tsp salt
- ½ tsp pepper

Directions:
1. Place rack in position 1 of the oven. Spray a 9-inch loaf pan with cooking spray.
2. In a large bowl, combine all ingredients until thoroughly mixed. Spread evenly in prepared pan.
3. Set oven to bake on 350°F for 45 minutes. After 5 minutes, place the pan in the oven and cook 40 minutes, or until top is golden brown. Slice and serve.
- **Nutrition Info:** Calories 169, Total Fat 5g, Saturated Fat 1g, Total Carbs 13g, Net Carbs 12g, Protein 18g, Sugar 3g, Fiber 1g, Sodium 540mg, Potassium 247mg, Phosphorus 202mg

223. Golden Beer-battered Cod

Servings: 4
Cooking Time: 15 Minutes
Ingredients:
- 2 eggs
- 1 cup malty beer
- 1 cup all-purpose flour
- ½ cup cornstarch
- 1 teaspoon garlic powder
- Salt and pepper, to taste
- 4 (4-ounce / 113-g) cod fillets
- Cooking spray

Directions:
1. In a shallow bowl, beat together the eggs with the beer. In another shallow bowl, thoroughly combine the flour and cornstarch. Sprinkle with the garlic powder, salt, and pepper.
2. Dredge each cod fillet in the flour mixture, then in the egg mixture. Dip each piece of fish in the flour mixture a second time.
3. Spritz the air fryer basket with cooking spray. Arrange the cod fillets in the pan in a single layer.

4. Put the air fryer basket on the baking pan and slide into Rack Position 2, select Air Fry, set temperature to 400ºF (205ºC), and set time to 15 minutes.
5. Flip the fillets halfway through the cooking time.
6. When cooking is complete, the cod should reach an internal temperature of 145ºF (63ºC) on a meat thermometer and the outside should be crispy. Let the fish cool for 5 minutes and serve.

224. Parmesan Fish With Pine Nuts

Servings: 4
Cooking Time: 15 Minutes
Ingredients:
- 2 tbsp fresh basil, chopped
- 2 garlic cloves, minced
- 2 tbsp olive oil
- 1 tbsp Parmesan cheese, grated
- salt and black pepper to taste
- 2 tbsp pine nuts
- 4 white fish fillets
- 2 tbsp olive oil

Directions:
1. Preheat Kalorik Maxx on Air Fry function to 350 F. Season the fish with salt and pepper. Place in the greased basket and fit in the baking tray. Cook the fillets for 8 minutes, flipping once. In a bowl, add basil, olive oil, pine nuts, garlic, and Parmesan cheese; mix well. Serve with the fish.

225. Citrus Cilantro Catfish

Servings: 2
Cooking Time: 20 Minutes
Ingredients:
- 2 catfish fillets
- 2 tsp blackening seasoning
- Juice of 1 lime
- 2 tbsp butter, melted
- 1 garlic clove, mashed
- 2 tbsp fresh cilantro, chopped

Directions:
1. In a bowl, blend garlic, lime juice, cilantro, and butter. Pour half of the mixture over the fillets and sprinkle with blackening seasoning. Place the fillets in the basket and press Start. Cook for 15 minutes at 360 F on AirFry function. Serve the fish topped with the remaining sauce.

226. Salmon Beans & Mushrooms

Servings: 6
Cooking Time: 25 Minutes
Ingredients:
- 4 salmon fillets
- 2 tbsp fresh parsley, minced
- 1/4 cup fresh lemon juice
- 1 tsp garlic, minced
- 1 tbsp olive oil
- 1/2 lb mushrooms, sliced
- 1/2 lb green beans, trimmed
- 1/2 cup parmesan cheese, grated
- Pepper
- Salt

Directions:
1. Fit the Kalorik Maxx oven with the rack in position
2. Heat oil in a small saucepan over medium-high heat.
3. Add garlic and sauté for 30 seconds.
4. Remove from heat and stir in lemon juice, parsley, pepper, and salt.
5. Arrange fish fillets, mushrooms, and green beans in baking pan and drizzle with oil mixture.
6. Sprinkle with grated parmesan cheese.
7. Set to bake at 400 F for 30 minutes. After 5 minutes place the baking pan in the preheated oven.
8. Serve and enjoy.
- **Nutrition Info:** Calories 225 Fat 11.5 g Carbohydrates 4.7 g Sugar 1.4 g Protein 27.5 g Cholesterol 58 mg

227. Roasted Nicoise Salad

Servings: 4
Cooking Time: 15 Minutes
Ingredients:
- 10 ounces (283 g) small red potatoes, quartered
- 8 tablespoons extra-virgin olive oil, divided
- 1 teaspoon kosher salt, divided
- ½ pound (227 g) green beans, trimmed
- 1 pint cherry tomatoes
- 1 teaspoon Dijon mustard
- 3 tablespoons red wine vinegar

- Freshly ground black pepper, to taste
- 1 (9-ounce / 255-g) bag spring greens, washed and dried if needed
- 2 (5-ounce / 142-g) cans oil-packed tuna, drained
- 2 hard-cooked eggs, peeled and quartered
- ⅓ cup kalamata olives, pitted

Directions:
1. In a large bowl, drizzle the potatoes with 1 tablespoon of olive oil and season with ¼ teaspoon of kosher salt. Transfer to the baking pan.
2. Slide the baking pan into Rack Position 2, select Roast, set temperature to 375ºF (190ºC), and set time to 15 minutes.
3. Meanwhile, in a mixing bowl, toss the green beans and cherry tomatoes with 1 tablespoon of olive oil and ¼ teaspoon of kosher salt until evenly coated.
4. After 10 minutes, remove the pan and fold in the green beans and cherry tomatoes. Return the pan to the oven and continue cooking.
5. Meanwhile, make the vinaigrette by whisking together the remaining 6 tablespoons of olive oil, mustard, vinegar, the remaining ½ teaspoon of kosher salt, and black pepper in a small bowl. Set aside.
6. When done, remove from the oven. Allow the vegetables to cool for 5 minutes.
7. Spread out the spring greens on a plate and spoon the tuna into the center of the greens. Arrange the potatoes, green beans, cheery tomatoes, and eggs around the tuna. Serve drizzled with the vinaigrette and scattered with the olives.

228. Baked Scallops

Servings: 4
Cooking Time: 15 Minutes
Ingredients:
- 1 lb scallops, frozen & thawed
- 1 tbsp garlic, grated
- 1/2 cup butter, melted
- 1 lemon, cut into wedges
- 1 tbsp olive oil
- Pepper
- Salt

Directions:
1. Fit the Kalorik Maxx oven with the rack in position
2. Add scallops and lemon into the baking dish and spread well.
3. Mix melted butter, oil, garlic, pepper, and salt and pour over scallops.
4. Set to bake at 400 F for 20 minutes. After 5 minutes place the baking dish in the preheated oven.
5. Serve and enjoy.

- **Nutrition Info:** Calories 341 Fat 27.4 g Carbohydrates 4.8 g Sugar 0.4 g Protein 19.6 g Cholesterol 98 mg

229. Buttery Crab Legs

Servings: 4
Cooking Time: 15 Minutes
Ingredients:
- 3 pounds crab legs
- 1 cup butter, melted

Directions:
1. Preheat Kalorik Maxx on AirFry function to 380 F. Dip the crab legs in salted water and let stay for a few minutes. Drain, pat dry, and place the legs in the basket and press Start. Cook for 10 minutes. Pour the butter over crab legs and serve.

230. Cheesy Tilapia Fillets

Servings: 4
Cooking Time: 15 Minutes
Ingredients:
- ¾ cup grated Parmesan cheese
- 1 tbsp olive oil
- 2 tsp paprika
- 1 tbsp chopped parsley
- ¼ tsp garlic powder
- 4 tilapia fillets

Directions:
1. Preheat Kalorik Maxx on Air Fry function to 350 F. Mix parsley, Parmesan cheese, garlic, and paprika in a bowl. Brush the olive oil over the fillets and then coat with the Parmesan mixture. Place the tilapia onto a lined baking sheet and cook for 8-10 minutes, turning once. Serve.

231. Cajun Salmon With Lemon

Servings: 1

Cooking Time: 10 Minutes
Ingredients:
- 1 salmon fillet
- ¼ tsp brown sugar
- Juice of ½ lemon
- 1 tbsp cajun seasoning
- 2 lemon wedges
- 1 tbsp fresh parsley, chopped

Directions:
1. Preheat Kalorik Maxx on Bake function to 350 F. Combine sugar and lemon and coat in the salmon. Sprinkle with the Cajun seasoning as well. Place a parchment paper on a baking tray and press Start. Cook for 14-16 minutes. Serve with lemon wedges and chopped parsley.

232. Sesame Seeds Coated Fish

Servings: 5
Cooking Time: 8 Minutes
Ingredients:
- 3 tablespoons plain flour
- 2 eggs
- ½ cup sesame seeds, toasted
- ½ cup breadcrumbs
- 1/8 teaspoon dried rosemary, crushed
- Pinch of salt
- Pinch of black pepper
- 3 tablespoons olive oil
- 5 frozen fish fillets (white fish of your choice)

Directions:
1. Preparing the Ingredients. In a shallow dish, place flour. In a second shallow dish, beat the eggs. In a third shallow dish, add remaining ingredients except fish fillets and mix till a crumbly mixture forms.
2. Coat the fillets with flour and shake off the excess flour.
3. Next, dip the fillets in the egg.
4. Then coat the fillets with sesame seeds mixture generously.
5. Preheat the Kalorik Maxx air fryer oven to 390 degrees F.
6. Air Frying. Line an Air fryer rack/basket with a piece of foil. Arrange the fillets into prepared basket.
7. Cook for about 14 minutes, flipping once after 10 minutes.

233. Spicy Halibut

Servings: 4
Cooking Time: 12 Minutes
Ingredients:
- 1 lb halibut fillets
- 1/2 tsp chili powder
- 1/2 tsp smoked paprika
- 1/4 cup olive oil
- 1/4 tsp garlic powder
- Pepper
- Salt

Directions:
1. Fit the Kalorik Maxx oven with the rack in position
2. Place halibut fillets in a baking dish.
3. In a small bowl, mix oil, garlic powder, paprika, pepper, chili powder, and salt.
4. Brush fish fillets with oil mixture.
5. Set to bake at 425 F for 17 minutes. After 5 minutes place the baking dish in the preheated oven.
6. Serve and enjoy.
- **Nutrition Info:** Calories 236 Fat 15.3 g Carbohydrates 0.5 g Sugar 0.1 g Protein 24 g Cholesterol 36 mg

234. Simple Lemon Salmon

Servings: 2
Cooking Time: 20 Minutes
Ingredients:
- 2 salmon fillets
- Salt to taste
- Zest of a lemon

Directions:
1. Spray the fillets with olive oil and rub them with salt and lemon zest. Line baking paper in a baking dish. Cook the fillets in your Kalorik Maxx for 10 minutes at 360 F on Air Fry, turning once.

MEATLESS RECIPES

235. Mushroom Club Sandwich

Servings: x
Cooking Time: x
Ingredients:
- ¼ tbsp. Worcestershire sauce
- ½ tsp. olive oil
- ½ flake garlic crushed
- ¼ cup chopped onion
- ¼ tbsp. red chili sauce
- ½ cup water
- 2 slices of white bread
- 1 tbsp. softened butter
- 1 cup minced mushroom
- 1 small capsicum

Directions:
1. Take the slices of bread and remove the edges. Now cut the slices horizontally.
2. Cook the ingredients for the sauce and wait till it thickens. Now, add the mushroom to the sauce and stir till it obtains the flavors. Roast the capsicum and peel the skin off. Cut the capsicum into slices. Apply the sauce on the slices.
3. Pre-heat the Kalorik Maxx oven for 5 minutes at 300 Fahrenheit. Open the basket of the Fryer and place the prepared Classic Sandwiches in it such that no two Classic Sandwiches are touching each other. Now keep the fryer at 250 degrees for around 15 minutes. Turn the Classic Sandwiches in between the cooking process to cook both slices. Serve the Classic Sandwiches with tomato ketchup or mint sauce.

236. Tofu, Carrot And Cauliflower Rice

Servings: 4
Cooking Time: 22 Minutes
Ingredients:
- ½ block tofu, crumbled
- 1 cup diced carrot
- ½ cup diced onions
- 2 tablespoons soy sauce
- 1 teaspoon turmeric
- Cauliflower:
- 3 cups cauliflower rice
- ½ cup chopped broccoli
- ½ cup frozen peas
- 2 tablespoons soy sauce
- 1 tablespoon minced ginger
- 2 garlic cloves, minced
- 1 tablespoon rice vinegar
- 1½ teaspoons toasted sesame oil

Directions:
1. Mix the tofu, carrot, onions, soy sauce, and turmeric in a baking pan and stir until well incorporated.
2. Slide the baking pan into Rack Position 2, select Roast, set temperature to 370ºF (188ºC) and set time to 10 minutes.
3. Flip the tofu and carrot halfway through the cooking time.
4. When cooking is complete, the tofu should be crisp.
5. Meanwhile, in a large bowl, combine all the ingredients for the cauliflower and toss well.
6. Remove the pan from the oven and add the cauliflower mixture to the tofu and stir to combine.
7. Return to the oven and set time to 12 minutes on Roast.
8. When cooking is complete, the vegetables should be tender.
9. Cool for 5 minutes before serving.

237. Green Chili Taquitos

Servings: 3
Cooking Time: 10 Minutes
Ingredients:
- Nonstick cooking spray
- 6 corn tortillas
- ¾ cup vegan cream cheese
- 1 cup vegan cheddar cheese, grated
- 4 oz. green chilies, diced & drained

Directions:
1. Place baking pan in position 2. Lightly spray fryer basket with cooking spray.
2. Wrap tortillas in paper towels and microwave 1 minute.
3. Spread the cream cheese over tortillas. Top with cheddar cheese and chilies. Roll up tightly. Place, seam side down, in fryer basket.

4. Place the basket on the baking pan and set oven to air fry on 350°F for 10 minutes or until tortillas are browned and crispy. Turn taquitos over halfway through cooking time. Serve immediately.
- **Nutrition Info:** Calories 706, Total Fat 34g, Saturated Fat 18g, Total Carbs 51g, Net Carbs 35g, Protein 24g, Sugar 11g, Fiber 16g, Sodium 2371mg, Potassium 1074mg, Phosphorus 850mg

238. Vegetable And Cheese Stuffed Tomatoes

Servings: 4
Cooking Time: 18 Minutes
Ingredients:
- 4 medium beefsteak tomatoes, rinsed
- ½ cup grated carrot
- 1 medium onion, chopped
- 1 garlic clove, minced
- 2 teaspoons olive oil
- 2 cups fresh baby spinach
- ¼ cup crumbled low-sodium feta cheese
- ½ teaspoon dried basil

Directions:
1. On your cutting board, cut a thin slice off the top of each tomato. Scoop out a ¼- to ½-inch-thick tomato pulp and place the tomatoes upside down on paper towels to drain. Set aside.
2. Stir together the carrot, onion, garlic, and olive oil in the baking pan.
3. Slide the baking pan into Rack Position 1, select Convection Bake, set temperature to 350ºF (180ºC) and set time to 5 minutes.
4. Stir the vegetables halfway through.
5. When cooking is complete, the carrot should be crisp-tender.
6. Remove from the oven and stir in the spinach, feta cheese, and basil.
7. Spoon ¼ of the vegetable mixture into each tomato and transfer the stuffed tomatoes to the oven. Set time to 13 minutes.
8. When cooking is complete, the filling should be hot and the tomatoes should be lightly caramelized.
9. Let the tomatoes cool for 5 minutes and serve.

239. Cilantro Roasted Carrots With Cumin Seeds

Servings: 4
Cooking Time: 15 Minutes
Ingredients:
- 1 lb carrots, julienned
- 1 tbsp olive oil
- 1 tsp cumin seeds
- 2 tbsp fresh cilantro, chopped

Directions:
1. Preheat Kalorik Maxx on AirFry function to 350 F. In a bowl, mix oil, carrots, and cumin seeds. Gently stir to coat the carrots well. Place the carrots in a baking tray and press Star. Cook for 10 minutes. Scatter fresh coriander over the carrots and serve.

240. Cheddar & Bean Burritos

Servings: 4
Cooking Time: 30 Minutes
Ingredients:
- 4 flour tortillas
- 1 cup grated cheddar cheese
- 1 (8 oz) can black beans, drained
- 1 tsp taco seasoning

Directions:
1. Preheat Kalorik Maxx on Bake function to 350 F. Mix the black beans with the taco seasoning. Divide the bean mixture between the tortillas and top with cheddar cheese. Roll the burritos and arrange them on a lined baking dish. Place in the oven and press Start. Cook for 5 minutes.

241. Fried Root Vegetable Medley With Thyme

Servings: 4
Cooking Time: 22 Minutes
Ingredients:
- 2 carrots, sliced
- 2 potatoes, cut into chunks
- 1 rutabaga, cut into chunks
- 1 turnip, cut into chunks
- 1 beet, cut into chunks
- 8 shallots, halved
- 2 tablespoons olive oil
- Salt and black pepper, to taste

- 2 tablespoons tomato pesto
- 2 tablespoons water
- 2 tablespoons chopped fresh thyme

Directions:
1. Toss the carrots, potatoes, rutabaga, turnip, beet, shallots, olive oil, salt, and pepper in a large mixing bowl until the root vegetables are evenly coated.
2. Place the root vegetables in the air fryer basket.
3. Put the air fryer basket on the baking pan and slide into Rack Position 2, select Air Fry, set temperature to 400ºF (205ºC) and set time to 22 minutes.
4. Stir the vegetables twice during cooking.
5. When cooking is complete, the vegetables should be tender.
6. Meanwhile, in a small bowl, whisk together the tomato pesto and water until smooth.
7. When ready, remove the root vegetables from the oven to a platter. Drizzle with the tomato pesto mixture and sprinkle with the thyme. Serve immediately.

242. Honey-glazed Roasted Veggies

Servings: 3 Cups
Cooking Time: 20 Minutes
Ingredients:
- Glaze:
- 2 tablespoons raw honey
- 2 teaspoons minced garlic
- ¼ teaspoon dried marjoram
- ¼ teaspoon dried basil
- ¼ teaspoon dried oregano
- ⅛ teaspoon dried sage
- ⅛ teaspoon dried rosemary
- ⅛ teaspoon dried thyme
- ½ teaspoon salt
- ¼ teaspoon ground black pepper
- Veggies:
- 3 to 4 medium red potatoes, cut into 1- to 2-inch pieces
- 1 small zucchini, cut into 1- to 2-inch pieces
- 1 small carrot, sliced into ¼-inch rounds
- 1 (10.5-ounce / 298-g) package cherry tomatoes, halved
- 1 cup sliced mushrooms
- 3 tablespoons olive oil

Directions:
1. Combine the honey, garlic, marjoram, basil, oregano, sage, rosemary, thyme, salt, and pepper in a small bowl and stir to mix well. Set aside.
2. Place the red potatoes, zucchini, carrot, cherry tomatoes, and mushroom in a large bowl. Drizzle with the olive oil and toss to coat.
3. Pour the veggies into the baking pan.
4. Slide the baking pan into Rack Position 2, select Roast, set temperature to 380ºF (193ºC) and set time to 15 minutes.
5. Stir the veggies halfway through.
6. When cooking is complete, the vegetables should be tender.
7. When ready, transfer the roasted veggies to the large bowl. Pour the honey mixture over the veggies, tossing to coat.
8. Spread out the veggies in the baking pan.
9. Increase the temperature to 390ºF (199ºC) and set time to 5 minutes on Roast.
10. When cooking is complete, the veggies should be tender and glazed. Serve warm.

243. Cheese With Spinach Enchiladas

Servings: 4
Cooking Time: 20 Minutes
Ingredients:
- 8 corn tortillas, warm
- 2 cups mozzarella cheese, shredded
- 1 cup ricotta cheese
- 1 cup spinach, torn
- 1 garlic clove, minced
- ½ cup sliced onions
- ½ cup sour cream
- 1 tbsp butter
- 1 can enchilada sauce

Directions:
1. Warm olive oil In a saucepan over medium heat and sauté garlic and onion for 3 minutes until soft. Stir in the spinach and cook for 5 more minutes until wilted. Remove from the heat and stir in the ricotta cheese, sour cream, and half of the mozzarella cheese.
2. Spoon ¼ cup of the spinach mixture in the middle of each tortilla. Roll up and place

seam side down in a baking dish. Pour the enchilada sauce over the tortillas and sprinkle with the remaining cheese. Cook in your Kalorik Maxx for 15 minutes at 380 F on Air Fry function.

244. Rosemary Butternut Squash Roast

Servings: 2
Cooking Time: 30 Minutes
Ingredients:
- 1 butternut squash
- 1 tbsp dried rosemary
- 2 tbsp maple syrup
- Salt to taste

Directions:
1. Place the squash on a cutting board and peel. Cut in half and remove the seeds and pulp. Slice into wedges and season with salt. Preheat Kalorik Maxx on Air Fry function to 350 F. Spray the wedges with cooking spray and sprinkle with rosemary. Place the wedges in the basket without overlapping and fit in the baking tray. Cook for 20 minutes, flipping once halfway through. Serve with maple syrup and goat cheese.

245. Potato Flat Cakes

Servings: x
Cooking Time: x
Ingredients:
- 2 or 3 green chilies finely chopped
- 1 ½ tbsp. lemon juice
- Salt and pepper to taste
- 2 tbsp. garam masala
- 2 cups sliced potato
- 3 tsp. ginger finely chopped
- 1-2 tbsp. fresh coriander leaves

Directions:
1. Mix the ingredients in a clean bowl and add water to it. Make sure that the paste is not too watery but is enough to apply on the potato slices.
2. Pre heat the Kalorik Maxx oven at 160 degrees Fahrenheit for 5 minutes. Place the French Cuisine Galettes in the fry basket and let them cook for another 25 minutes at the same temperature. Keep rolling them over to get a uniform cook. Serve either with mint sauce or ketchup.

246. Cottage Cheese Fried Baked Pastry

Servings: x
Cooking Time: x
Ingredients:
- 1 or 2 green chilies that are finely chopped or mashed
- ½ tsp. cumin
- 1 tsp. coarsely crushed coriander
- 1 dry red chili broken into pieces
- A small amount of salt (to taste)
- ½ tsp. dried mango powder
- ½ tsp. red chili power
- 1-2 tbsp. coriander
- 2 tbsp. unsalted butter
- 1 ½ cup all-purpose flour
- A pinch of salt to taste
- Water
- 2 cups mashed cottage cheese
- ¼ cup boiled peas
- 1 tsp. powdered ginger

Directions:
1. Mix the dough for the outer covering and make it stiff and smooth. Leave it to rest in a container while making the filling.
2. Cook the ingredients in a pan and stir them well to make a thick paste. Roll the paste out.
3. Roll the dough into balls and flatten them. Cut them in halves and add the filling. Use water to help you fold the edges to create the shape of a cone.
4. Pre-heat the Kalorik Maxx oven for around 5 to 6 minutes at 300 Fahrenheit. Place all the samosas in the fry basket and close the basket properly. Keep the Kalorik Maxx oven at 200 degrees for another 20 to 25 minutes. Around the halfway point, open the basket and turn the samosas over for uniform cooking. After this, fry at 250 degrees for around 10 minutes in order to give them the desired golden-brown color. Serve hot. Recommended sides are tamarind or mint sauce.

247. Roasted Butternut Squash With Maple Syrup

Servings: 4
Cooking Time: 30 Minutes
Ingredients:
- 1 lb butternut squash
- 1 tsp dried rosemary
- 2 tbsp maple syrup
- Salt to taste

Directions:
1. Place the squash on a cutting board and peel. Cut in half and remove the seeds and pulp. Slice into wedges and season with salt. Spray with cooking spray and sprinkle with rosemary.
2. Preheat Kalorik Maxx on AirFry function to 350 F. Transfer the wedges to the greased basket without overlapping. Press Start and cook for 20 minutes. Serve drizzled with maple syrup.

248. Teriyaki Tofu

Servings: 3
Cooking Time: 15 Minutes
Ingredients:
- Nonstick cooking spray
- 14 oz. firm or extra firm tofu, pressed & cut in 1-inch cubes
- ¼ cup cornstarch
- ½ tsp salt
- ½ tsp ginger
- ½ tsp white pepper
- 3 tbsp. olive oil
- 12 oz. bottle vegan teriyaki sauce

Directions:
1. Lightly spray baking pan with cooking spray.
2. In a shallow dish, combine cornstarch, salt, ginger, and pepper.
3. Heat oil in a large skillet over med-high heat.
4. Toss tofu cubes in cornstarch mixture then add to skillet. Cook 5 minutes, turning over halfway through, until tofu is nicely seared. Transfer the tofu to the prepared baking pan.
5. Set oven to convection bake on 350°F for 15 minutes.
6. Pour all but ½ cup teriyaki sauce over tofu and stir to coat. After oven has preheated for 5 minutes, place the baking pan in position 2 and bake tofu 10 minutes.
7. Turn tofu over, spoon the sauce in the pan over it and bake another 10 minutes. Serve with reserved sauce for dipping.
- **Nutrition Info:** Calories 469, Total Fat 25g, Saturated Fat 4g, Total Carbs 33g, Net Carbs 30g, Protein 28g, Sugar 16g, Fiber 3g, Sodium 2424mg, Potassium 571mg, Phosphorus 428mg

249. Crispy Tofu Sticks

Servings: 4
Cooking Time: 14 Minutes
Ingredients:
- 2 tablespoons olive oil, divided
- ½ cup flour
- ½ cup crushed cornflakes
- Salt and black pepper, to taste
- 14 ounces (397 g) firm tofu, cut into ½-inch-thick strips

Directions:
1. Grease the air fryer basket with 1 tablespoon of olive oil.
2. Combine the flour, cornflakes, salt, and pepper on a plate.
3. Dredge the tofu strips in the flour mixture until they are completely coated. Transfer the tofu strips to the greased basket.
4. Drizzle the remaining 1 tablespoon of olive oil over the top of tofu strips.
5. Put the air fryer basket on the baking pan and slide into Rack Position 2, select Air Fry, set temperature to 360ºF (182ºC), and set time to 14 minutes.
6. Flip the tofu strips halfway through the cooking time.
7. When cooking is complete, the tofu strips should be crispy. Remove from the oven and serve warm.

250. Korean Tempeh Steak With Broccoli

Servings: 4
Cooking Time: 15 Minutes + Marinating Time
Ingredients:
- 16 oz tempeh, cut into 1 cm thick pieces

- 1 pound broccoli, cut into florets
- ⅓ cup fermented soy sauce
- 2 tbsp sesame oil
- ⅓ cup sherry
- 1 tsp soy sauce
- 1 tsp white sugar
- 1 tsp cornstarch
- 1 tbsp olive oil
- 1 garlic clove, minced

Directions:
1. In a bowl, mix cornstarch, sherry, fermented soy sauce, sesame oil, soy sauce, sugar, and tempeh pieces. Marinate for 45 minutes.
2. Then, add in garlic, olive oil, and ginger. Place in the basket and fit in the baking tray; cook for 10 minutes at 390 F on Air Fry function, turning once halfway through. Serve.

251. Cauliflower Rice With Tofu & Peas

Servings: 4
Cooking Time: 30 Minutes
Ingredients:
- Tofu:
- ½ block tofu, crumbled
- ½ cup diced onion
- 2 tbsp soy sauce
- 1 tsp turmeric
- 1 cup diced carrot
- Cauliflower:
- 3 cups cauliflower rice
- 2 tbsp soy sauce
- ½ cup chopped broccoli
- 2 garlic cloves, minced
- 1 ½ tsp toasted sesame oil
- 1 tbsp minced ginger
- ½ cup frozen peas
- 1 tbsp rice vinegar

Directions:
1. Preheat Kalorik Maxx on Air Fry function to 370 F. Combine all the tofu ingredients in a greased baking dish. Cook for 10 minutes.
2. Meanwhile, place all cauliflower ingredients in a large bowl and mix to combine. Stir the cauliflower mixture in the tofu baking dish and return to the oven; cook for 12 minutes. Serve.

252. Spicy Thai-style Vegetables

Servings: 4
Cooking Time: 8 Minutes
Ingredients:
- 1 small head Napa cabbage, shredded, divided
- 1 medium carrot, cut into thin coins
- 8 ounces (227 g) snow peas
- 1 red or green bell pepper, sliced into thin strips
- 1 tablespoon vegetable oil
- 2 tablespoons soy sauce
- 1 tablespoon sesame oil
- 2 tablespoons brown sugar
- 2 tablespoons freshly squeezed lime juice
- 2 teaspoons red or green Thai curry paste
- 1 serrano chile, deseeded and minced
- 1 cup frozen mango slices, thawed
- ½ cup chopped roasted peanuts or cashews

Directions:
1. Put half the Napa cabbage in a large bowl, along with the carrot, snow peas, and bell pepper. Drizzle with the vegetable oil and toss to coat. Spread them evenly in the air fryer basket.
2. Put the air fryer basket on the baking pan and slide into Rack Position 2, select Roast, set temperature to 375ºF (190ºC), and set time to 8 minutes.
3. Meanwhile, whisk together the soy sauce, sesame oil, brown sugar, lime juice, and curry paste in a small bowl.
4. When done, the vegetables should be tender and crisp. Remove from the oven and put the vegetables back into the bowl. Add the chile, mango slices, and the remaining cabbage. Pour over the dressing and toss to coat. Top with the roasted nuts and serve.

253. Spicy Kung Pao Tofu

Servings: 4
Cooking Time: 10 Minutes
Ingredients:
- ⅓ cup Asian-Style sauce
- 1 teaspoon cornstarch

- ½ teaspoon red pepper flakes, or more to taste
- 1 pound (454 g) firm or extra-firm tofu, cut into 1-inch cubes
- 1 small carrot, peeled and cut into ¼-inch-thick coins
- 1 small green bell pepper, cut into bite-size pieces
- 3 scallions, sliced, whites and green parts separated
- 3 tablespoons roasted unsalted peanuts

Directions:
1. In a large bowl, whisk together the sauce, cornstarch, and red pepper flakes. Fold in the tofu, carrot, pepper, and the white parts of the scallions and toss to coat. Spread the mixture evenly in the baking pan.
2. Slide the baking pan into Rack Position 2, select Roast, set temperature to 375ºF (190ºC), and set time to 10 minutes.
3. Stir the ingredients once halfway through the cooking time.
4. When done, remove from the oven. Serve sprinkled with the peanuts and scallion greens.

254.Chili Veggie Skewers

Servings: 4
Cooking Time: 20 Minutes
Ingredients:
- 2 tbsp cornflour
- 1 cup canned white beans, drained
- ⅓ cup grated carrots
- 2 boiled and mashed potatoes
- ¼ cup chopped fresh mint leaves
- ½ tsp garam masala powder
- ½ cup paneer
- 1 green chili
- 1-inch piece of fresh ginger
- 3 garlic cloves
- Salt to taste

Directions:
1. Preheat Kalorik Maxx on Air Fry function to 390 F. Place the beans, carrots, garlic, ginger, chili, paneer, and mint in a food processor; process until smooth. Transfer to a bowl. Add in the mashed potatoes, cornflour, salt, and garam masala powder and mix until fully incorporated.
2. Divide the mixture into 12 equal pieces. Shape each of the pieces around a skewer. Cook in your Kalorik Maxx for 10 minutes, turning once. Serve.

255.Cottage Cheese And Mushroom Mexican Burritos

Servings:x
Cooking Time:x
Ingredients:
- ½ cup mushrooms thinly sliced
- 1 cup cottage cheese cut in too long and slightly thick Oregano Fingers
- A pinch of salt to taste
- ½ tsp. red chili flakes
- 1 tsp. freshly ground peppercorns
- ½ cup pickled jalapenos
- 1-2 lettuce leaves shredded.
- ½ cup red kidney beans (soaked overnight)
- ½ small onion chopped
- 1 tbsp. olive oil
- 2 tbsp. tomato puree
- ¼ tsp. red chili powder
- 1 tsp. of salt to taste
- 4-5 flour tortillas
- 1 or 2 spring onions chopped finely. Also cut the greens.
- Take one tomato. Remove the seeds and chop it into small pieces.
- 1 green chili chopped.
- 1 cup of cheddar cheese grated.
- 1 cup boiled rice (not necessary).
- A few flour tortillas to put the filing in.

Directions:
1. Cook the beans along with the onion and garlic and mash them finely.
2. Now, make the sauce you will need for the burrito. Ensure that you create a slightly thick sauce.
3. For the filling, you will need to cook the ingredients well in a pan and ensure that the vegetables have browned on the outside.
4. To make the salad, toss the ingredients together. Place the tortilla and add a layer of sauce, followed by the beans and the filling

at the center. Before you roll it, you will need to place the salad on top of the filling.
5. Pre-heat the Kalorik Maxx oven for around 5 minutes at 200 Fahrenheit. Open the fry basket and keep the burritos inside. Close the basket properly. Let the Air
6. Fryer remain at 200 Fahrenheit for another 15 minutes or so. Halfway through, remove the basket and turn all the burritos over in order to get a uniform cook.

256. Veg Momo's Recipe

Servings: x
Cooking Time: x
Ingredients:
- 2 tsp. ginger-garlic paste
- 2 tsp. soya sauce
- 2 tsp. vinegar
- 1 ½ cup all-purpose flour
- ½ tsp. salt or to taste
- 5 tbsp. water
- 2 cup carrots grated
- 2 cup cabbage grated
- 2 tbsp. oil

Directions:
1. Squeeze the dough and cover it with plastic wrap and set aside. Next, cook the ingredients for the filling and try to ensure that the vegetables are covered well with the sauce.
2. Roll the dough and cut it into a square. Place the filling in the center. Now, wrap the dough to cover the filling and pinch the edges together.
3. Pre heat the Kalorik Maxx oven at 200° F for 5 minutes. Place the gnocchi's in the fry basket and close it. Let them cook at the same temperature for another 20 minutes. Recommended sides are chili sauce or ketchup.

257. Gourd French Cuisine Galette

Servings: x
Cooking Time: x
Ingredients:
- 2 or 3 green chilies finely chopped
- 1 ½ tbsp. lemon juice
- Salt and pepper to taste
- 2 tbsp. garam masala
- 2 cups sliced gourd
- 1 ½ cup coarsely crushed peanuts
- 3 tsp. ginger finely chopped
- 1-2 tbsp. fresh coriander leaves

Directions:
1. Mix the ingredients in a clean bowl.
2. Mold this mixture into round and flat French Cuisine Galettes.
3. Wet the French Cuisine Galettes slightly with water. Coat each French Cuisine Galette with the crushed peanuts.
4. Pre heat the Kalorik Maxx oven at 160 degrees Fahrenheit for 5 minutes. Place the French Cuisine Galettes in the fry basket and let them cook for another 25 minutes at the same temperature. Keep rolling them over to get a uniform cook. Serve either with mint sauce or ketchup

258. Paprika Cauliflower

Servings: 4
Cooking Time: 20 Minutes
Ingredients:
- 1 large head cauliflower, broken into small florets
- 2 teaspoons smoked paprika
- 1 teaspoon garlic powder
- Salt and freshly ground black pepper, to taste
- Cooking spray

Directions:
1. Spray the air fryer basket with cooking spray.
2. In a medium bowl, toss the cauliflower florets with the smoked paprika and garlic powder until evenly coated. Sprinkle with salt and pepper.
3. Place the cauliflower florets in the basket and lightly mist with cooking spray.
4. Put the air fryer basket on the baking pan and slide into Rack Position 2, select Air Fry, set temperature to 400ºF (205ºC), and set time to 20 minutes.
5. Stir the cauliflower four times during cooking.
6. Remove the cauliflower from the oven and serve hot.

259. Russian-style Eggplant Caviar

Servings: 3
Cooking Time: 20 Minutes
Ingredients:
- 3 medium eggplants
- ½ red onion, chopped and blended
- 2 tbsp balsamic vinegar
- 1 tbsp olive oil
- Salt to taste

Directions:
1. Arrange the eggplants on the AirFryer basket and fit in the baking tray. Cook them in your Kalorik Maxx for 15 minutes at 380 F on Bake function. Let cool.
2. Peel the cooled eggplants and chop them. Process the onion and eggplant in a blender. Add in the vinegar, olive oil, and salt, then blend again. Serve cool with bread and tomato sauce.

260. Lemony Brussels Sprouts And Tomatoes

Servings: 4
Cooking Time: 20 Minutes
Ingredients:
- 1 pound (454 g) Brussels sprouts, trimmed and halved
- 1 tablespoon extra-virgin olive oil
- Sea Salt and freshly ground black pepper, to taste
- ½ cup sun-dried tomatoes, chopped
- 2 tablespoons freshly squeezed lemon juice
- 1 teaspoon lemon zest

Directions:
1. Line the air fryer basket with aluminum foil.
2. Toss the Brussels sprouts with the olive oil in a large bowl. Sprinkle with salt and black pepper.
3. Spread the Brussels sprouts in a single layer in the basket.
4. Put the air fryer basket on the baking pan and slide into Rack Position 2, select Roast, set temperature to 400ºF (205ºC), and set time to 20 minutes.
5. When done, the Brussels sprouts should be caramelized. Remove from the oven to a serving bowl, along with the tomatoes, lemon juice, and lemon zest. Toss to combine. Serve immediately.

261. Parmesan Breaded Zucchini Chips

Servings: 5
Cooking Time: 20 Minutes
Ingredients:
- For the zucchini chips:
- 2 medium zucchini
- 2 eggs
- ⅓ cup bread crumbs
- ⅓ cup grated Parmesan cheese
- Salt
- Pepper
- Cooking oil
- For the lemon aioli:
- ½ cup mayonnaise
- ½ tablespoon olive oil
- Juice of ½ lemon
- 1 teaspoon minced garlic
- Salt
- Pepper

Directions:
1. Preparing the Ingredients. To make the zucchini chips:
2. Slice the zucchini into thin chips (about ⅛ inch thick) using a knife or mandoline.
3. In a small bowl, beat the eggs. In another small bowl, combine the bread crumbs, Parmesan cheese, and salt and pepper to taste.
4. Spray the Oven rack/basket with cooking oil.
5. Dip the zucchini slices one at a time in the eggs and then the bread crumb mixture. You can also sprinkle the bread crumbs onto the zucchini slices with a spoon.
6. Place the zucchini chips in the Oven rack/basket, but do not stack. Place the Rack on the middle-shelf of the Kalorik Maxx air fryer oven.
7. Air Frying. Cook in batches. Spray the chips with cooking oil from a distance (otherwise, the breading may fly off). Cook for 10 minutes.
8. Remove the cooked zucchini chips from the air fryer oven, then repeat step 5 with the remaining zucchini.

9. To make the lemon aioli:
10. While the zucchini is cooking, combine the mayonnaise, olive oil, lemon juice, and garlic in a small bowl, adding salt and pepper to taste. Mix well until fully combined.
11. Cool the zucchini and serve alongside the aioli.
- **Nutrition Info:** CALORIES: 192; FAT: 13G; PROTEIN: 6

262. Okra Flat Cakes

Servings:x
Cooking Time:x
Ingredients:
- 2 or 3 green chilies finely chopped
- 1 ½ tbsp. lemon juice
- Salt and pepper to taste
- 2 tbsp. garam masala
- 2 cups sliced okra
- 3 tsp. ginger finely chopped
- 1-2 tbsp. fresh coriander leaves

Directions:
1. Mix the ingredients in a clean bowl and add water to it. Make sure that the
2. paste is not too watery but is enough to apply on the okra.
3. Pre heat the Kalorik Maxx oven at 160 degrees Fahrenheit for 5 minutes. Place the French Cuisine Galettes in the fry basket and let them cook for another 25 minutes at the same temperature. Keep rolling them over to get a uniform cook. Serve either with mint sauce or ketchup.

263. Potato Fried Baked Pastry

Servings:x
Cooking Time:x
Ingredients:
- 1 tsp. powdered ginger
- 1 or 2 green chilies that are finely chopped or mashed
- ½ tsp. cumin
- 1 tsp. coarsely crushed coriander
- 1 dry red chili broken into pieces
- A small amount of salt (to taste)
- 2 tbsp. unsalted butter
- 1 ½ cup all-purpose flour
- A pinch of salt to taste
- Add as much water as required to make the dough stiff and firm
- 2-3 big potatoes boiled and mashed
- ¼ cup boiled peas
- ½ tsp. dried mango powder
- ½ tsp. red chili power.
- 1-2 tbsp. coriander.

Directions:
1. Mix the dough for the outer covering and make it stiff and smooth. Leave it to rest in a container while making the filling. Cook the ingredients in a pan and stir them well to make a thick paste. Roll the paste out.
2. Roll the dough into balls and flatten them. Cut them in halves and add the filling. Use water to help you fold the edges to create the shape of a cone. Pre-heat the Kalorik Maxx oven for around 5 to 6 minutes at 300 Fahrenheit.
3. Place all the samosas in the fry basket and close the basket properly. Keep the Kalorik Maxx oven at 200 degrees for another 20 to 25 minutes. Around the halfway point, open the basket and turn the samosas over for uniform cooking. After this, fry at 250 degrees for around 10 minutes in order to give them the desired golden-brown color. Serve hot. Recommended sides are tamarind or mint sauce.

264. Zucchini Crisps

Servings:4
Cooking Time: 25 Minutes
Ingredients:
- 4 small zucchinis, cut lengthwise
- ½ cup Parmesan cheese, grated
- ½ cup breadcrumbs
- ¼ cup butter, melted
- ¼ cup fresh parsley, chopped
- 4 garlic cloves, minced
- Salt and black pepper to taste

Directions:
1. Preheat Kalorik Maxx on AirFry function to 350 F. In a bowl, mix breadcrumbs, Parmesan cheese, garlic, and parsley. Season with salt and pepper and stir in the butter.

2. Arrange the zucchinis with the cut side up. Spread the cheese mixture onto the zucchini and place them in the basket. Press Start and cook for 14-16 minutes. Serve hot.

265. Honey-glazed Baby Carrots

Servings: 4
Cooking Time: 12 Minutes
Ingredients:
- 1 pound (454 g) baby carrots
- 2 tablespoons olive oil
- 1 tablespoon honey
- 1 teaspoon dried dill
- Salt and black pepper, to taste

Directions:
1. Place the carrots in a large bowl. Add the olive oil, honey, dill, salt, and pepper and toss to coat well.
2. Transfer the carrots to the air fryer basket.
3. Put the air fryer basket on the baking pan and slide into Rack Position 2, select Roast, set temperature to 350ºF (180ºC), and set time to 12 minutes.
4. Stir the carrots once during cooking.
5. When cooking is complete, the carrots should be crisp-tender. Remove from the oven and serve warm.

266. Grandma´s Ratatouille

Servings: 2
Cooking Time: 30 Minutes
Ingredients:
- 1 tbsp olive oil
- 3 Roma tomatoes, thinly sliced
- 2 garlic cloves, minced
- 1 zucchini, thinly sliced
- 2 yellow bell peppers, sliced
- 1 tbsp vinegar
- 2 tbsp herbs de Provence
- Salt and black pepper to taste

Directions:
1. Preheat Kalorik Maxx on AirFry function to 390 F. Place all ingredients in a bowl. Season with salt and pepper and stir to coat. Arrange the vegetable on a baking dish and place in the Kalorik Maxx oven. Cook for 15 minutes, shaking occasionally. Let sit for 5 more minutes after the timer goes off.

267. Cabbage Flat Cakes

Servings: x
Cooking Time: x
Ingredients:
- 2 or 3 green chilies finely chopped
- 1 ½ tbsp. lemon juice
- Salt and pepper to taste
- 2 tbsp. garam masala
- 2 cups halved cabbage leaves
- 3 tsp. ginger finely chopped
- 1-2 tbsp. fresh coriander leaves

Directions:
1. Mix the ingredients in a clean bowl and add water to it. Make sure that the paste is not too watery but is enough to apply on the cabbage.
2. Pre heat the Kalorik Maxx oven at 160 degrees Fahrenheit for 5 minutes. Place the French Cuisine Galettes in the fry basket and let them cook for another 25 minutes at the same temperature. Keep rolling them over to get a uniform cook. Serve either with mint sauce or ketchup.

268. Mint French Cuisine Galette

Servings: x
Cooking Time: x
Ingredients:
- 1-2 tbsp. fresh coriander leaves
- 2 or 3 green chilies finely chopped
- 1 ½ tbsp. lemon juice
- Salt and pepper to taste
- 2 cups mint leaves (Sliced fine)
- 2 medium potatoes boiled and mashed
- 1 ½ cup coarsely crushed peanuts
- 3 tsp. ginger finely chopped

Directions:
1. Mix the sliced mint leaves with the rest of the ingredients in a clean bowl.
2. Mold this mixture into round and flat French Cuisine Galettes.
3. Wet the French Cuisine Galettes slightly with water. Coat each French Cuisine Galette with the crushed peanuts.
4. Pre heat the Kalorik Maxx oven at 160 degrees Fahrenheit for 5 minutes. Place the French Cuisine Galettes in the fry basket

and let them cook for another 25 minutes at the same temperature. Keep rolling them over to get a uniform cook. Serve either with mint sauce or ketchup.

269. Banana Best Homemade Croquette

Servings: x
Cooking Time: x
Ingredients:
- 2 tsp. garam masala
- 4 tbsp. chopped coriander
- 3 tbsp. cream
- 3 tbsp. chopped capsicum
- 3 eggs
- 2 ½ tbsp. white sesame seeds
- 2 cups sliced banana
- 3 onions chopped
- 5 green chilies-roughly chopped
- 1 ½ tbsp. ginger paste
- 1 ½ tsp. garlic paste
- 1 ½ tsp. salt
- 3 tsp. lemon juice

Directions:
1. Grind the ingredients except for the egg and form a smooth paste. Coat the banana in the paste. Now, beat the eggs and add a little salt to it.
2. Dip the coated bananas in the egg mixture and then transfer to the sesame seeds and coat the vegetables well. Place the vegetables on a stick.
3. Pre heat the Kalorik Maxx oven at 160 degrees Fahrenheit for around 5 minutes. Place the sticks in the basket and let them cook for another 25 minutes at the same temperature. Turn the sticks over in between the cooking process to get a uniform cook.

270. Onion Rings

Servings: 4
Cooking Time: 10 Minutes
Ingredients:
- 1 large spanish onion
- 1/2 cup buttermilk
- 2 eggs, lightly beaten
- 3/4 cups unbleached all-purpose flour
- 3/4 cups panko bread crumbs
- 1/2 teaspoon baking powder
- 1/2 teaspoon Cayenne pepper, to taste
- Salt

Directions:
1. Preparing the Ingredients. Start by cutting your onion into 1/2 thick rings and separate. Smaller pieces can be discarded or saved for other recipes.
2. Beat the eggs in a large bowl and mix in the buttermilk, then set it aside.
3. In another bowl combine flour, pepper, bread crumbs, and baking powder.
4. Use a large spoon to dip a whole ring in the buttermilk, then pull it through the flour mix on both sides to completely coat the ring.
5. Air Frying. Cook about 8 rings at a time in your Kalorik Maxx air fryer oven for 8-10 minutes at 360 degrees shaking half way through.
- **Nutrition Info:** CALORIES: 225; FAT: 3.8G; PROTEIN:19G; FIBER:2.4G

271. Chili Sweet Potato Fries

Servings: 4
Cooking Time: 30 Minutes
Ingredients:
- ½ tsp salt
- ½ tsp garlic powder
- ½ tsp chili powder
- ¼ tsp ground cumin
- 3 tbsp olive oil
- 3 sweet potatoes, cut into thick strips

Directions:
1. In a bowl, mix salt, garlic powder, chili powder, and cumin, and whisk in oil. Coat in the potato strips and arrange them on the basket, without overcrowding. Press Start and cook for 20-25 minutes at 380 F on AirFry function or until crispy. Serve hot.

272. Cheesy Spinach Toasties

Servings: x
Cooking Time: x
Ingredients:
- 1 tsp. coarsely crushed green chilies
- 2 tbsp. grated pizza cheese
- 1 cup milk

- 2 toasted bread slices cut into triangles
- 1 tbsp. butter
- 1 tbsp. all-purpose flour
- 1 small onion finely chopped
- 1-2 flakes garlic finely chopped
- Half a bunch of spinach that has been boiled and crushed (does not have to be crushed finely)
- 1 tbsp. fresh cream
- Some salt and pepper to taste

Directions:
1. Take a pan and melt some butter in it. Also add some onions and garlic.
2. Now keep roasting them in the butter until the onions are caramelized or attain a golden-brown color.
3. Into this pan add the required amount of all-purpose flour. Continue to roast for 3 minutes or so. Add milk and keep stirring until you bring it to a boil.
4. Add green chilies, cream, spinach and seasoning. Mix the ingredients properly and let it cook until the mixture thickens. Toast some bread. Apply the paste made in the previous step on the bread.
5. Sprinkle some grated cheese on top of the paste.
6. Pre heat the Kalorik Maxx oven at 290 Fahrenheit for around 4 minutes. Put the toasts in the Fry basket and let it continue to cook for another 10 minutes at the same temperature.

273. Parmesan Cabbage With Blue Cheese Sauce

Servings: 4
Cooking Time: 25 Minutes
Ingredients:
- ½ head cabbage, cut into wedges
- 2 cups Parmesan cheese, chopped
- 4 tbsp butter, melted
- Salt and black pepper to taste
- ½ cup blue cheese sauce

Directions:
1. Drizzle cabbage wedges with butter and coat with Parmesan cheese. Place them in the frying basket and cook for 20 minutes at 380 F on AirFry setting. Serve topped with blue cheese sauce.

SNACKS AND DESSERTS RECIPES

274. Vanilla Peanut Butter Cake

Servings: 8
Cooking Time: 30 Minutes
Ingredients:
- 1 1/2 cups all-purpose flour
- 1/3 cup vegetable oil
- 1 tsp baking soda
- 1/2 cup peanut butter powder
- 1 tsp vanilla
- 1 tbsp apple cider vinegar
- 1 cup of water
- 1 cup of sugar
- 1/2 tsp salt

Directions:
1. Fit the Kalorik Maxx oven with the rack in position
2. In a large mixing bowl, mix together flour, baking soda, peanut butter powder, sugar, and salt.
3. In a small bowl, whisk together oil, vanilla, vinegar, and water.
4. Pour oil mixture into the flour mixture and stir until well combined.
5. Pour batter into the greased cake pan.
6. Set to bake at 350 F for 35 minutes. After 5 minutes place the cake pan in the preheated oven.
7. Slice and serve.
- **Nutrition Info:** Calories 264 Fat 1.8 g Carbohydrates 43.2 g Sugar 25.3 g Protein 2.6 g Cholesterol 0 mg

275. Almond Cranberry Muffins

Servings: 6
Cooking Time: 30 Minutes
Ingredients:
- 2 eggs
- 1 tsp vanilla
- 1/4 cup sour cream
- 1/2 cup cranberries
- 1 1/2 cups almond flour
- 1/4 tsp cinnamon
- 1 tsp baking powder
- 1/4 cup Swerve
- Pinch of salt

Directions:
1. Fit the Kalorik Maxx oven with the rack in position
2. Line 6-cups muffin tin with cupcake liners and set aside.
3. In a bowl, beat sour cream, vanilla, and eggs.
4. Add remaining ingredients except for cranberries and beat until smooth.
5. Add cranberries and fold well.
6. Pour batter into the prepared muffin tin.
7. Set to bake at 325 F for 30 minutes. After 5 minutes place muffin tin in the preheated oven.
8. Serve and enjoy.
- **Nutrition Info:** Calories 218 Fat 16 g Carbohydrates 18 g Sugar 10 g Protein 8 g Cholesterol 59 mg

276. Cinnamon Apple Crisp

Servings: 4
Cooking Time: 35 Minutes
Ingredients:
- 1/8 tsp ground clove
- 1/8 tsp ground nutmeg
- 2 tbsp honey
- 4 1/2 cups apples, diced
- 1 tsp ground cinnamon
- 1 tbsp cornstarch
- 1 tsp vanilla
- 1/2 lemon juice
- For topping:
- 1 cup rolled oats
- 1/3 cup coconut oil, melted
- 1 tsp cinnamon
- 1/3 cup honey
- 1/2 cup almond flour

Directions:
1. Fit the Kalorik Maxx oven with the rack in position
2. In a medium bowl, mix apples, vanilla, lemon juice, and honey. Sprinkle spices and cornstarch on top and stir well.
3. Pour apple mixture into the greased baking dish.

4. In a small bowl, mix together coconut oil, cinnamon, almond flour, oats, and honey and spread on top of apple mixture.
5. Set to bake at 350 F for 40 minutes. After 5 minutes place the baking dish in the preheated oven.
6. Serve and enjoy.
- **Nutrition Info:** Calories 450 Fat 21 g Carbohydrates 65 g Sugar 40 g Protein 4 g Cholesterol 0 mg

277. Pita Bread Cheese Pizza

Servings: 4
Cooking Time: 6 Minutes
Ingredients:
- 1 pita bread
- ¼ cup Mozzarella cheese
- 7 slices pepperoni
- ¼ cup sausage
- 1 tablespoon yellow onion, sliced thinly
- 1 tablespoon pizza sauce
- 1 drizzle extra-virgin olive oil
- ½ teaspoon fresh garlic, minced

Directions:
1. Preheat the Air fryer to 350 degree F and grease an Air fryer basket.
2. Spread pizza sauce on the pita bread and add sausages, pepperoni, onions, garlic and cheese.
3. Drizzle with olive oil and place it in the Air fryer basket.
4. Cook for about 6 minutes and dish out to serve warm.
- **Nutrition Info:** Calories: 56, Fat: 3.6g, Carbohydrates: 6.7g, Sugar: 3.6g, Protein: 0.3g, Sodium: 0mg

278. Seafood Turnovers

Servings: x
Cooking Time: x
Ingredients:
- ½ teaspoon dried dill weed
- 1 sheet frozen puff pastry, thawed
- 1 egg yolk, beaten
- 1 tablespoon water
- 1 (6-ounce) can small shrimp, drained
- ½ cup ricotta cheese
- 3 green onions, finely chopped
- 1 cup shredded Havarti cheese

Directions:
1. In medium bowl, combine shrimp, ricotta, green onions, Havarti, and dill weed and mix well.
2. Gently roll puff pastry into 12-inch by 18-inch rectangle. Cut into 24 3-inch squares. Place 2 teaspoons shrimp mixture in center of each square. Beat egg yolk with water in small bowl. Brush edges of pastry with egg yolk mixture. Fold puff pastry over filling, forming triangles; press edges with fork to seal.
3. Flash freeze turnovers in single layer on baking sheet. Then pack in rigid containers, with waxed paper separating the layers. Label containers and freeze.
4. To reheat: Preheat oven to 450ºF. Place frozen turnovers on baking sheet. Bake at 450ºF for 4 minutes; then turn oven down to 400ºF and bake for 12 to 15 minutes longer or until pastry is golden and filling is hot.

279. Margherita Pizza

Servings: 4
Cooking Time: 18 Minutes
Ingredients:
- 1 whole-wheat pizza crust
- 1/2 cup mozzarella cheese, grated
- 1/2 cup can tomatoes
- 2 tbsp olive oil
- 3 Roma tomatoes, sliced
- 10 basil leaves

Directions:
1. Fit the Kalorik Maxx oven with the rack in position
2. Roll out whole wheat pizza crust using a rolling pin. Make sure the crust is ½-inch thick.
3. Sprinkle olive oil on top of pizza crust.
4. Spread can tomatoes over pizza crust.
5. Arrange sliced tomatoes and basil on pizza crust. Sprinkle grated cheese on top.
6. Place pizza on top of the oven rack and set to bake at 425 F for 23 minutes.
7. Slice and serve.

- **Nutrition Info:** Calories 126 Fat 7.9 g Carbohydrates 11.3 g Sugar 4.2 g Protein 3.6 g Cholesterol 2 mg

280. Tasty Jalapeno Poppers

Servings: 4
Cooking Time: 13 Minutes
Ingredients:
- 4 jalapeno peppers, slice in half and deseeded
- 4 oz goat cheese, crumbled
- 1/4 tsp chili powder
- 2 tbsp chunky salsa
- Pepper
- Salt

Directions:
1. Fit the Kalorik Maxx oven with the rack in position 2.
2. In a small bowl, mix together cheese, chunky salsa, chili powder, pepper, and salt.
3. Stuff cheese mixture into each jalapeno half and place in the air fryer basket then place the air fryer basket in the baking pan.
4. Place a baking pan on the oven rack. Set to air fry at 350 F for 13 minutes.
5. Serve and enjoy.
- **Nutrition Info:** Calories 68 Fat 5.1 g Carbohydrates 2.5 g Sugar 1.6 g Protein 3.6 g Cholesterol 20 mg

281. Deep-dish Giant Double Chocolate Chip Cookie

Servings: x
Cooking Time: x
Ingredients:
- 1 large egg
- 1 cup all-purpose flour
- ½ tsp baking powder
- ½ tsp salt
- 1 cup chocolate chip
- ½ cup unsalted butter
- ½ cup light brown sugar
- ½ cup white sugar
- 1 tsp vanilla
- ½ cup chocolate chunks

Directions:
1. Preheat oven to 350°F.
2. Melt butter in Kalorik Maxx oven over low heat.
3. Add sugars and stir well.
4. Incorporate vanilla and egg, and beat quickly to make sure eggs do not cook.
5. Stir in flour, baking soda and salt.
6. Fold in chocolate chips and chunks and spread dough out in Kalorik Maxx oven lightly with a spatula to flatten.
7. Bake for 25 minutes until cookie appears browned on top.

282. Cappuccino Blondies

Servings: 16
Cooking Time: 30 Minutes
Ingredients:
- Nonstick cooking spray
- 1 cup butter, soft
- 2 cups brown sugar
- 2 eggs
- 2 tsp baking powder
- 1 tsp salt
- 4 tsp espresso powder
- 2 2/3 cups flour

Directions:
1. Place rack in position Lightly spray an 8x11-inch baking pan with cooking spray.
2. In a large bowl, beat together butter and sugar. Add eggs and beat until light and fluffy.
3. Add baking powder, salt, and espresso and mix well. Stir in flour until combined.
4. Set oven to bake on 350°F for 35 minutes.
5. Spread batter in prepared pan. Once oven has preheated, place brownies in oven and bake 25-30 minutes.
6. Remove from oven and let cool before cutting.
- **Nutrition Info:** Calories 296, Total Fat 12g, Saturated Fat 7g, Total Carbs 44g, Net Carbs 43g, Protein 3g, Sugar 28g, Fiber 1g, Sodium 254mg, Potassium 137mg, Phosphorus 82mg

283. Tasty Potato Wedges

Servings: 4
Cooking Time: 15 Minutes
Ingredients:

- 2 medium potatoes, cut into wedges
- 1/4 tsp garlic powder
- 1/4 tsp pepper
- 1/2 tsp paprika
- 1 1/2 tbsp olive oil
- 1/8 tsp cayenne
- 1 tsp sea salt

Directions:
1. Fit the Kalorik Maxx oven with the rack in position 2.
2. Soak potato wedges into the water for 30 minutes.
3. Drain well and pat dry with a paper towel.
4. In a bowl, toss potato wedges with remaining ingredients.
5. Place potato wedges in the air fryer basket then place an air fryer basket in the baking pan.
6. Place a baking pan on the oven rack. Set to air fry at 400 F for 15 minutes.
7. Serve and enjoy.
- **Nutrition Info:** Calories 120 Fat 5.4 g Carbohydrates 17.1 g Sugar 1.3 g Protein 1.9 g Cholesterol 0 mg

284. Italian Rice Balls

Servings: 8 Rice Balls
Cooking Time: 10 Minutes
Ingredients:
- 1½ cups cooked sticky rice
- ½ teaspoon Italian seasoning blend
- ¾ teaspoon salt, divided
- 8 black olives, pitted
- 1 ounce (28 g) Mozzarella cheese, cut into tiny pieces (small enough to stuff into olives)
- 2 eggs
- ⅓ cup Italian bread crumbs
- ¾ cup panko bread crumbs
- Cooking spray

Directions:
1. Stuff each black olive with a piece of Mozzarella cheese.
2. In a bowl, combine the cooked sticky rice, Italian seasoning blend, and ½ teaspoon of salt and stir to mix well. Form the rice mixture into a log with your hands and divide it into 8 equal portions. Mold each portion around a black olive and roll into a ball.
3. Transfer to the freezer to chill for 10 to 15 minutes until firm.
4. In a shallow dish, place the Italian bread crumbs. In a separate shallow dish, whisk the eggs. In a third shallow dish, combine the panko bread crumbs and remaining salt.
5. One by one, roll the rice balls in the Italian bread crumbs, then dip in the whisked eggs, finally coat them with the panko bread crumbs.
6. Arrange the rice balls in the air fryer basket and spritz both sides with cooking spray.
7. Put the air fryer basket on the baking pan and slide into Rack Position 2, select Air Fry, set temperature to 390ºF (199ºC), and set time to 10 minutes.
8. Flip the balls halfway through the cooking time.
9. When cooking is complete, the rice balls should be golden brown. Remove from the oven and serve warm.

285. Flavorful Coconut Cake

Servings: 8
Cooking Time: 20 Minutes
Ingredients:
- 5 eggs, separated
- 1/2 cup erythritol
- 1/4 cup coconut milk
- 1/2 cup coconut flour
- 1/2 tsp baking powder
- 1/2 tsp vanilla
- 1/2 cup butter softened
- Pinch of salt

Directions:
1. Fit the Kalorik Maxx oven with the rack in position
2. Grease cake pan with butter and set aside.
3. In a bowl, beat sweetener and butter until combined.
4. Add egg yolks, coconut milk, and vanilla and mix well.
5. Add baking powder, coconut flour, and salt and stir well.
6. In another bowl, beat egg whites until stiff peak forms.

7. Gently fold egg whites into the cake mixture.
8. Pour batter in a prepared cake pan.
9. Set to bake at 400 F for 25 minutes. After 5 minutes place the cake pan in the preheated oven.
10. Slice and serve.
- **Nutrition Info:** Calories 84 Fat 5.9 g Carbohydrates 4.2 g Sugar 0.6 g Protein 4 g Cholesterol 102 mg

286. Strawberries Stew

Servings: 4
Cooking Time: 20 Minutes
Ingredients:
- 1-pound strawberries, halved
- 4 tablespoons stevia
- 1 tablespoon lemon juice
- 1 and ½ cups water

Directions:
1. In a pan that fits your air fryer, mix all the ingredients, toss, put it in the fryer and cook at 340 degrees F for 20 minutes.
2. Divide the stew into cups and serve cold.
- **Nutrition Info:** calories 176, fat 2, fiber 1, carbs 3, protein 5

287. Coffee Flavored Doughnuts

Servings: 6
Cooking Time: 6 Minutes
Ingredients:
- Coconut sugar, ¼ cup
- White all-purpose flour, 1 cup
- Baking powder, 1 tsp.
- Salt, ½ tsp.
- Sunflower oil, 1 tbsp.
- Coffee, ¼ cup
- Aquafaba, 2 tbsps.

Directions:
1. Combine the sugar, flour, baking powder, salt in a mixing bowl.
2. In another bowl, combine the aquafaba, sunflower oil, and coffee.
3. Mix to form a dough.
4. Let the dough rest inside the fridge.
5. Preheat the air fryer to 4000 F.
6. Knead the dough and create doughnuts.
7. Arrange inside the air fryer in single layer and cook for 6 minutes.

8. Do not shake so that the donut maintains its shape.
- **Nutrition Info:** Calories: 113 Protein: 2.16g Fat: 2.54g Carbs: 20.45g

288. Nutella Banana Pastries

Servings: 4
Cooking Time: 12 Minutes
Ingredients:
- 1 puff pastry sheet
- ½ cup Nutella
- 2 bananas, peeled and sliced

Directions:
1. Cut the pastry sheet into 4 equal-sized squares.
2. Spread the Nutella on each square of pastry evenly.
3. Divide the banana slices over Nutella.
4. Fold each square into a triangle and with wet fingers, slightly press the edges.
5. Then with a fork, press the edges firmly.
6. Press "Power Button" of Air Fry Oven and turn the dial to select the "Air Fry" mode.
7. Press the Time button and again turn the dial to set the cooking time to 12 minutes.
8. Now push the Temp button and rotate the dial to set the temperature at 375 degrees F.
9. Press "Start/Pause" button to start.
10. When the unit beeps to show that it is preheated, open the lid.
11. Arrange the pastries in greased "Air Fry Basket" and insert in the oven.
12. Serve warm.
- **Nutrition Info:** Calories 221 Total Fat 10 g Saturated Fat 2.7 g Cholesterol 26 mg Sodium 103 mg Total Carbs 31.6 g Fiber 2.6 g Sugar 14.4 g Protein 3.4 g

289. Simple Lemon Pie

Servings: 8
Cooking Time: 45 Minutes
Ingredients:
- 3 eggs
- 3.5 oz butter, melted
- 3 lemon juice
- 1 lemon zest, grated
- 4 oz erythritol
- 5.5 oz almond flour

- Salt

Directions:
1. Fit the Kalorik Maxx oven with the rack in position
2. In a bowl, mix together butter, 1 oz sweetener, 3 oz almond flour, and salt.
3. Transfer the dough in a pie dish and spread evenly and bake for 20 minutes.
4. In a separate bowl, mix together eggs, lemon juice, lemon zest, remaining flour, sweetener, and salt.
5. Pour egg mixture on prepared crust.
6. Set to bake at 350 F for 35 minutes. After 5 minutes place the pie dish in the preheated oven.
7. Slice and serve.
- **Nutrition Info:** Calories 229 Fat 21.5 g Carbohydrates 5.3 g Sugar 1.4 g Protein 6.5 g Cholesterol 88 mg

290. Buffalo Style Cauliflower

Servings: x
Cooking Time: x
Ingredients:
- ¼ cup Frank's red-hot sauce
- 1 Tbsp fresh lime juice
- Chopped parsley or cilantro
- 2 Tbsp olive oil
- 1 head cauliflower
- Salt and pepper, to taste
- 2 Tbsp unsalted butter

Directions:
1. Preheat oven to 375°F.
2. Chop off tough flower part at the base of the cauliflower. Break into
3. small to medium sized florets.
4. In a microwave-safe bowl, melt butter.
5. Add hot sauce and lime juice to butter and stir.
6. Heat Kalorik Maxx oven to medium-low heat.
7. Add oil and cauliflower florets. Saute until nicely browned, 4-5 minutes.
8. Pour in hot sauce mixture and stir to coat evenly.
9. Place in oven for 15-20 minutes, until cauliflower is softened.
10. Remove from oven and sprinkle with parsley or cilantro.

291. Spicy Snack Mix

Servings: x
Cooking Time: x
Ingredients:
- ½ cup butter, melted
- 3 tablespoons Worcestershire sauce
- 2 teaspoons dried Italian seasoning
- ½ teaspoon crushed red pepper flakes
- 2 cups salted mixed nuts
- 2 cups small pretzels
- 2 cups potato sticks
- teaspoon white pepper

Directions:
1. Preheat oven to 300ºF. Pour nuts, pretzels, and potato sticks onto two cookie sheets with sides. In small saucepan, combine melted butter with remaining ingredients. Drizzle over the nut mixture. Toss to coat. Bake at 300ºF for 20 to 25 minutes, or until mixture is glazed and fragrant, stirring once during baking.
2. Cool snack mix and pack into zipper-lock bags. Label bags and freeze.
3. To thaw and reheat: Thaw at room temperature for 1 to 3 hours. Spread on baking sheet and reheat in 300ºF oven for 5 to 8 minutes, until crisp.

292. Easy Lemon Cheesecake

Servings: 8
Cooking Time: 55 Minutes
Ingredients:
- 4 eggs
- 2 tbsp swerve
- 1 fresh lemon juice
- 18 oz ricotta cheese
- 1 fresh lemon zest

Directions:
1. Fit the Kalorik Maxx oven with the rack in position
2. In a large bowl, beat ricotta cheese until smooth.
3. Add egg one by one and whisk well.
4. Add lemon juice, lemon zest, and swerve and mix well.

5. Transfer mixture into the greased cake pan.
6. Set to bake at 350 F for 60 minutes. After 5 minutes place the cake pan in the preheated oven.
7. Slice and serve.
- **Nutrition Info:** Calories 122 Fat 7.3 g Carbohydrates 4.2 g Sugar 0.5 g Protein 10.1 g Cholesterol 102 mg

293. Baked Yoghurt

Servings: x
Cooking Time: x
Ingredients:
- 1 cup blackberries
- Handful of mint leaves
- 3 tsp. sugar
- 4 tsp. water
- 2 cups condensed milk
- 2 cups yoghurt
- 2 cups fresh cream
- 1 cup fresh strawberries
- 1 cup fresh blueberries

Directions:
1. Mix the ingredients together and create a thick mixture. Transfer this into baking bowls ensuring that you do not overfill.
2. Preheat the fryer to 300 Fahrenheit for five minutes. You will need to place the bowls in the basket and cover it. Cook it for fifteen minutes. When you shake the bowls, the mixture should just shake but not break. Leave it in the refrigerator to set and then arrange the fruits, garnish and serve.

294. Easy Blueberry Muffins

Servings: 12
Cooking Time: 30 Minutes
Ingredients:
- 5.5 oz plain yogurt
- ½ cup fresh blueberries
- 2 tsp baking powder, gluten-free
- ¼ cup Swerve
- 2 ½ cups almond flour
- ½ tsp vanilla
- 3 eggs
- Pinch of salt

Directions:
1. Fit the Kalorik Maxx oven with the rack in position
2. Line 6-cups muffin tin with cupcake liners and set aside.
3. In a bowl, whisk egg, yogurt, vanilla, and salt until smooth.
4. Add flour, swerve and baking powder and blend again until smooth.
5. Add blueberries and stir well.
6. Pour batter into the prepared muffin tin.
7. Set to bake at 325 F for 35 minutes. After 5 minutes place muffin tin in the preheated oven.
8. Serve and enjoy.
- **Nutrition Info:** Calories 63 Fat 4.2 g Carbohydrates 3.6 g Sugar 1.8 g Protein 3.4 g Cholesterol 42 mg

295. Easy Bacon Jalapeno Poppers

Servings: 10
Cooking Time: 8 Minutes
Ingredients:
- 10 jalapeno peppers, cut in half and remove seeds
- 1/3 cup cream cheese, softened
- 1/4 tsp paprika
- 1/4 tsp chili powder
- 5 bacon strips, cut in half

Directions:
1. Fit the Kalorik Maxx oven with the rack in position 2.
2. In a small bowl, mix cream cheese, paprika, chili powder, and bacon and stuff in each jalapeno half.
3. Place jalapeno half in the air fryer basket then place an air fryer basket in the baking pan.
4. Place a baking pan on the oven rack. Set to air fry at 370 F for 8 minutes.
5. Serve and enjoy.
- **Nutrition Info:** Calories 83 Fat 7.4 g Carbohydrates 1.3 g Sugar 0.5 g Protein 2.8 g Cholesterol 9 mg

296. Tasty Broccoli Fritters

Servings: 4
Cooking Time: 30 Minutes
Ingredients:

- 3 cups broccoli florets, steam & chopped
- 2 eggs, lightly beaten
- 2 garlic cloves, minced
- 2 cups cheddar cheese, shredded
- 1/4 cup breadcrumbs
- 1/2 tsp Italian seasoning
- Pepper
- Salt

Directions:
1. Fit the Kalorik Maxx oven with the rack in position
2. Add all ingredients into the large bowl and mix until well combined.
3. Make patties from broccoli mixture and place in baking pan.
4. Set to bake at 375 F for 35 minutes. After 5 minutes place the baking pan in the preheated oven.
5. Serve and enjoy.
- **Nutrition Info:** Calories 313 Fat 21.7 g Carbohydrates 10.9 g Sugar 2.1 g Protein 19.8 g Cholesterol 142 mg

297. Cheesy Baked Potatoes

Servings: 6
Cooking Time: 20 Minutes
Ingredients:
- 12 small red potatoes
- 1 teaspoon kosher salt, divided
- 1 tablespoon extra-virgin olive oil
- ¼ cup grated sharp Cheddar cheese
- ¼ cup sour cream
- 2 tablespoons chopped chives
- 2 tablespoons grated Parmesan cheese

Directions:
1. Add the potatoes to a large bowl. Sprinkle with the ½ teaspoon of the salt and drizzle with the olive oil. Toss to coat. Place the potatoes in the baking pan.
2. Slide the baking pan into Rack Position 2, select Roast, set temperature to 375ºF (190ºC) and set time to 15 minutes.
3. When cooking is complete, remove the pan and let the potatoes rest for 5 minutes. Halve the potatoes lengthwise. Using a spoon, scoop the flesh into a bowl, leaving a thin shell of skin. Arrange the potato halves in the pan.
4. Mash the potato flesh until smooth. Stir in the remaining ½ teaspoon of the salt, Cheddar cheese, sour cream and chives. Transfer the filling into a pastry bag with one corner snipped off. Pipe the filling into the potato shells, mounding up slightly. Sprinkle with the Parmesan cheese.
5. Select Roast, set temperature to 375ºF (190ºC) and set time to 5 minutes.
6. When cooking is complete, the tops should be browning slightly. Remove from the oven and let the potatoes cool slightly before serving.

298. Tasty Gingersnap Cookies

Servings: 8
Cooking Time: 10 Minutes
Ingredients:
- 1 egg
- 1/2 tsp ground cinnamon
- 1/2 tsp ground ginger
- 1 tsp baking powder
- 3/4 cup erythritol
- 1/2 tsp vanilla
- 1/8 tsp ground cloves
- 1/4 tsp ground nutmeg
- 2/4 cup butter, melted
- 1 1/2 cups almond flour
- Pinch of salt

Directions:
1. Fit the Kalorik Maxx oven with the rack in position
2. In a mixing bowl, mix together all dry ingredients.
3. In another bowl, mix together all wet ingredients.
4. Add dry ingredients to the wet ingredients and mix until a dough-like mixture is formed.
5. Cover and place in the refrigerator for 30 minutes.
6. Make cookies from dough and place onto a parchment-lined baking pan.
7. Set to bake at 350 F for 15 minutes. After 5 minutes place the baking pan in the preheated oven.
8. Serve and enjoy.

- **Nutrition Info:** Calories 142 Fat 14.7 g Carbohydrates 1.8 g Sugar 0.3 g Protein 2 g Cholesterol 51 mg

299. Almond Flour Blackberry Muffins

Servings: 8
Cooking Time: 12 Minutes
Ingredients:
- ½ cup fresh blackberries
- Dry Ingredients:
- 1½ cups almond flour
- 1 teaspoon baking powder
- ½ teaspoon baking soda
- ½ cup Swerve
- ¼ teaspoon kosher salt
- Wet Ingredients:
- 2 eggs
- ¼ cup coconut oil, melted
- ½ cup milk
- ½ teaspoon vanilla paste

Directions:
1. Line an 8-cup muffin tin with paper liners.
2. Thoroughly combine the almond flour, baking powder, baking soda, Swerve, and salt in a mixing bowl.
3. Whisk together the eggs, coconut oil, milk, and vanilla in a separate mixing bowl until smooth.
4. Add the wet mixture to the dry and fold in the blackberries. Stir with a spatula just until well incorporated.
5. Spoon the batter into the prepared muffin cups, filling each about three-quarters full.
6. Put the muffin tin into Rack Position 1, select Convection Bake, set temperature to 350ºF (180ºC), and set time to 12 minutes.
7. When done, the tops should be golden and a toothpick inserted in the middle should come out clean.
8. Allow the muffins to cool in the muffin tin for 10 minutes before removing and serving

300. Cheesy Zucchini Tots

Servings: 8
Cooking Time: 6 Minutes
Ingredients:
- 2 medium zucchini (about 12 ounces / 340 g), shredded
- 1 large egg, whisked
- ½ cup grated pecorino romano cheese
- ½ cup panko bread crumbs
- ¼ teaspoon black pepper
- 1 clove garlic, minced
- Cooking spray

Directions:
1. Using your hands, squeeze out as much liquid from the zucchini as possible. In a large bowl, mix the zucchini with the remaining ingredients except the oil until well incorporated.
2. Make the zucchini tots: Use a spoon or cookie scoop to place tablespoonfuls of the zucchini mixture onto a lightly floured cutting board and form into 1-inch logs.
3. Spritz the air fryer basket with cooking spray. Place the zucchini tots in the pan.
4. Put the air fryer basket on the baking pan and slide into Rack Position 2, select Air Fry, set temperature to 375ºF (190ºC), and set time to 6 minutes.
5. When cooking is complete, the tots should be golden brown. Remove from the oven to a serving plate and serve warm.

CPSIA information can be obtained
at www.ICGtesting.com
Printed in the USA
LVHW061159050223
738710LV00028B/512